Veterinary Ocular Emergencies

Commissioning editor: Mary Seager
Development editor: Caroline Savage
Production controller: Anthony Read
Desk editor: Jackie Holding
Cover designer: Alan Studholme

Veterinary Ocular Emergencies

David L Williams MA VetMB PhD CertVOphthal MRCVS

Department of Clinical Veterinary Medicine, University of Cambridge, Madingley Road, Cambridge CB3 OES, UK

Kathy Barrie DVM DipACVO

Animal Eye Clinic, Sunshine Animal Hospital, 8008 West Waters Avenue, Tampa, Florida, USA

Thomas Ffrangcon Evans DVM MRCVS

Hospital for Small Animals, The Royal (Dick) School of Veterinary Studies, University of Edinburgh, Midlothian EH25 9RG, UK

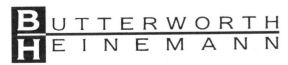

OXFORD   AUCKLAND   BOSTON   JOHANNESBURG   MELBOURNE   NEW DELHI

Butterworth-Heinemann
An imprint of Elsevier Science
Linacre House, Jordan Hill, Oxford OX2 8DP
225 Wildwood Avenue, Woburn, MA 01801-2041

First published 2002

British Library Cataloguing in Publication Data
Williams, David L.
    Veterinary ocular emergencies
    1. Veterinary ophthalmology   2. Veterinary emergencies
    I Title   II. Barrie, Kathy   III. Evans, Thomas Ffrangcon
    636'.08977'026

Library of Congress Cataloging in Publication Data
A catalog record of this book is available from the Library of Congress

ISBN 0 7506 3560 6

Medical knowledge is constantly changing. As new information becomes
available, changes in treatment, procedures, equipment and the use of drugs
become necessary. The authors and the publishers have taken care to ensure
that the information given in this text is accurate and up to date. However,
readers are strongly advised to confirm that the information, especially with
regard to drug usage, complies with the latest legislation and standards of
practice.

Composition by Scribe Design, Gillingham, Kent, UK
Printed and bound in Great Britain by MPG Books Ltd, Bodmin, Cornwall

Contents

Preface

All too many veterinarians leave veterinary college with little exposure to ophthalmic cases and certainly next to no experience of even the most common ocular emergencies. Veterinary colleges generally admit referral cases, and so even when ophthalmology is well taught as a major core curriculum subject there is little opportunity to see ocular emergencies which are dealt with in first-opinion settings. This book is designed as a helping hand to all practitioners who are presented with an ocular emergency having had little introduction, either theoretical or practical, to veterinary ophthalmology or especially to ocular emergencies.

The book is not designed, however, to do away with the need for referral consultation in a specialist centre. If it is considered that the ocular disorder for which the animal is presented may be serious, with ocular pain or potential blindness, a referral or second opinion should always be offered to the client. Many pets are insured and it is to the benefit of the animal, the owner and yourself to have a second opinion on the case.

The eye is without doubt a special structure and vision is, some would say, a veritable miracle and a delicate one at that. Surgery of the eye, in particular, should always involve sensitive tissue handling with plenty of irrigating fluid. Cadaver practice prior to one's first surgical enterprise is essential. But the eye is not holy, not an organ which can only be dealt with by specialists. The aim of this volume is to allow veterinarians in general practice to deal better with emergencies which would otherwise result in pain and/or blindness. Thus our ultimate hope is that the book will improve the treatment of animals presented, as well as helping the vets who treat these animals to feel better-equipped to diagnose and treat these often difficult cases.

Thomas Evans 2002

Introduction

Some may consider that there are quite enough veterinary ophthalmic texts on the market at present – why do we need another? We suggest that there are two specific problems with the current texts, excellent and comprehensive as they are. The first is that to find diagnostic and therapeutic strategies in an emergency is almost impossible. Most texts require at least an evening's read to distil out the necessary diagnostic features and treatment requirements for a specific emergency condition be it a surgical condition at the ocular surface, such as a staphyloma (see Appendix B for the Ocular dictionary), or a predominantly medical condition in the posterior segment such as a sudden total retinal detachment.

Secondly, most texts are presented with an anatomical breakdown of ocular conditions. The animal does not, however, present as if saying 'I have a problem with my iridocorneal angle,' but rather 'I have a red eye' or 'I am suddenly blind'. Thus to be useful an emergency text needs to be thoroughly problem-oriented, not an easy task given a structure such as the eye which is so neatly packaged anatomically.

This text aims to fill that gap in the market in four ways. A problem-based first part will give the basics on diagnostic signs such as the red eye, the painful eye or the blind eye. That is where to start in assessing an ocular emergency. Secondly, each ocular emergency is discussed with regard to diagnostic tests applicable and therapeutic regimes advised.

Thirdly, both of these first two areas are heavily illustrated not by pictures: these can be found in the growing number of excellent atlases being produced by Barnett (1990), Barnett *et al.* (1995), Crispin and Barnett (1997) and Walde (1990); but by diagrams demonstrating the plan of attack in both the diagnostic work up of a case and the treatment regimen to be used. Fourthly, the authors feel that veterinarians are much better placed to deal with an emergency when knowing a reasonable amount of the basic science background behind the pathogenesis of ocular damage and the mechanisms underlying successful treatment. Therefore, while the text gives diagnostic and therapeutic suggestions including step-by-step flow diagrams, it also discusses the background to the disease processes and the ameliorating effects of treatment.

Reading through the whole text sequentially, one may be struck by a number of repetitions: these are unavoidable to ensure that each section has the opportunity to stand on its own when read in an emergency situation. It is hoped, however, that having the same information presented in different contexts throughout the text will be helpful in aiding understanding and remembering facts rather than be annoying and repetitious. The aim of this book is to provide a useful starting point in an emergency situation where the step-by-step diagram and table format allow rapid appreciation of important information. Also, once the emergency is over, it will be possible to read the discussion sections at leisure to elucidate some of the basic science background. In this way, should the same type of emergency arise again, it will be possible to approach it with a greater degree of understanding both regarding pathogenic mechanisms and therapeutic rationale.

We have attempted to write the portions for background reading in a style which is easy and enjoyable to read. Some may find this annoying and prefer a more scientific and less familiar manner. Given the number of texts in densely written scientific prose we have sought not to use that approach, and hope that readers will find this text easy to use both in the emergency situation and also for reading once the emergency has been resolved.

Chapter 1 touches on the diagnostic principles and techniques in dealing with an emergency; Chapter 2 looks as the various commonly presented conditions associated with problems with the eye; while Chapters 3 to 10 cover the initial diagnosis and treatment. Three appendices are also provided. Appendix A deals with the common applied diagnostic methods. This section is not included in the main text as some veterinary surgeons may find it common knowledge while others will find a thorough description of instruments such as a Schiotz tonometer useful. Appendix B is a veterinary ophthalmic dictionary. As ophthalmic nomenclature is very specialized all specific words mentioned in the text are explained in this section of the handbook. Appendix C is a drug index, where we have tried to include most of the drugs (human as well as veterinary) that are used for treatment of eye diseases in animals.

One final criticism is likely, perhaps not from general veterinary surgeons but from our colleagues in specialist practice. They will say, with perhaps some justification, that in general practice one does not need to know the ins and outs of treatment of uveitis or glaucoma cases. Such animals, they will say, need referring to a specialist trained in dealing with the sort of ophthalmic nightmares considered in this book. This may well be the case, and some specialists may even feel done out of a job if the diagnostic protocols and therapeutic regimens used are set out in detail. We feel, however, that such an approach would be short sighted and in the best interests of nobody, let alone the animal itself. Even when the specialist practice is only a car ride away, and the owners are happy to pay, the referring veterinarian must be able to define that referral is needed and give immediate treatment in every situation. In many cases distance, financial considerations or the time delay between presentation and an emergency referral means that it is up to the veterinarian to give care for the emergency case through the short term and often for longer. And who knows – perhaps dealing in this way with a few such cases, with the help of this book, will attract you further into the fascinating world of veterinary ophthalmology, leading you to train to be one of those specialists. Nevertheless the authors understand that many of these cases are, in the normal run of events, better referred immediately to a specialist. Situations where this is the case are marked thus ® in the text: referral is recommended in these cases.

It may be argued that most of the paragraphs here are preceded by an ®. Obviously, as veterinarians earning our living from ophthalmic referrals we are hardly going to dissuade you from asking for a second opinion, are we! Most cases will benefit from a referral, yet the whole point of this book is to equip veterinary surgeons with the knowledge to give immediate treatment that is appropriate, to recognize cases requiring referral and, in cases where referral is not appropriate, to make the best diagnostic and therapeutic interventions possible.

Chapter 1

Diagnostic principles and techniques

1.1 Performing an ocular examination in an emergency situation

The temptation, in an emergency, is to abandon the standard ophthalmic examination which would be undertaken under normal circumstances and merely concentrate on the immediately obvious ocular signs. Thus, in a dog with an eyelid laceration the globe is only cursorily examined. Given a cat with a corneal ulcer, the lids and intra-ocular structures are ignored. This failure to perform a standard examination will, in many if not the majority of cases, result in failure either fully to reach the correct diagnosis or to identify important, but less obvious, concurrent ocular disease or damage. In the dog mentioned above there may be a globe rupture as well as the eyelid laceration. In the cat the corneal pathology may be related to a post-traumatic eyelid defect with trichiasis while the corneal lesion may cause reflex miosis or more pronounced uveitis. In the first case failure to appreciate concurrent disease could result in loss of the eye, while in the second the rushed examination misses both the cause of the presenting sign and the potentially important intra-ocular sequelae.

Thus, a systematic approach is vital to every emergency ocular examination, as shown in Box 1.1. The evaluation should begin with an assessment of vision using the menace and startle responses, and then determination of pupil size and pupillary light response, including the swinging light test to detect functional optic nerve defects. The examination of the eye itself starts with distant direct ophthalmoscopy. This calms the animal rather than beginning the examination with one's head close to the animal's muzzle. It allows evaluation of pupil size and any opacity of the ocular media. Next the eyelids and adnexa, including the conjunctiva, are examined with the direct ophthalmoscope at a setting of +20 D. Remember that the conjunctiva is found covering the globe (bulbar conjunctiva) and the inner aspect of the eyelid (palpebral conjunctiva). Thus while uveitis or glaucoma affect the vasculature of the globe alone, conjunctivitis involves the vessels of the bulbar and palpebral conjunctiva. In assessing the conjunctiva both surfaces of the nictitating membrane should be examined as should the conjunctiva right to the depths of the fornices. This may be done later, after topical anaesthesia and fixing the margin of the third eyelid with a pair of haemostats or Babcock forceps, everting and looking behind the third eyelid. Next, in order, the cornea, anterior chamber, iris, lens, vitreous, retina and optic nerve head are examined with the dioptre settings of the direct ophthalmoscope at from +20 D (cornea and sclera) and +10 D (iris and lens) to 0 D (retina).

After full examination, ancillary aids should be brought into play. We consider that, given the simplicity of the test, every animal presenting as an ocular emergency

1 Assessment of vision:
Menace response
Dazzle response
Pupillary light reflex
Swinging light test

2 Distant direct ophthalmoscopy:
Assess pupil size and symmetry
Assess clarity of ocular media

3 Adnexa:
Lids
Conjunctiva
Nictitating membrane
Nasolacrimal system

4 Cornea:
Transparency   +20 D
Structural integrity

5 Uvea:
Colour   +10 D
Contour

6 Lens:
Transparency   +10 D ± 5 D
Position
Stability

7 Vitreous and retina:
Position
Tapetal reflectivity 0 ± 3 D
Vascular system

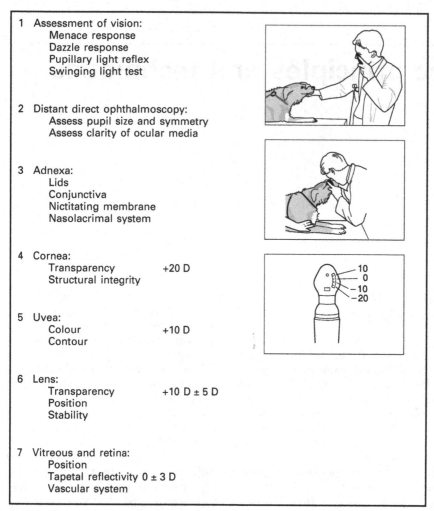

Box 1.1 Routine ophthalmological examination

should have a Schirmer I tear test performed (Appendix A). Measurement of intra-ocular pressure by applanation tonometry is more difficult given the expense of tonometers such as the Tonopen, but on the other hand the purchase of a Schiotz tonometer is well within the budget of a practice keen to provide an adequate ophthalmic work up. The importance of early diagnosis of raised intra-ocular pressure, and of following treatment response in animals with glaucoma, renders it almost essential that every practice has access to at least a Schiotz tonometer (details of using the Schiotz to optimal effect are given in Appendix A).

1.2 Recording observations made in an ocular emergency

The ophthalmic emergency might seem the least appropriate time to make detailed notes and drawings of the ocular signs presented. However, if one is already in the habit of carefully recording what one sees at an ophthalmic examination, this is tremendously useful for two reasons. First, it is important to have written and diagrammatic records of what was seen at presentation, in order better to be able to monitor the progress and hopefully the recovery of ocular health. Secondly, recording observations and particularly drawing annotated diagrams tend to improve one's assessment of lesions in the eye and ensure that small lesions have not been missed. In the ophthalmic emergency it is, however, important to be able to record ocular signs quickly and to have a ready method of diagrammatically noting signs in such a way as to differentiate, for instance, between corneal oedema, infiltration and scarring or a retinal haemorrhage, cellular infiltrate or a small area of retinal detachment. Two useful papers have been produced in the human ophthalmic literature suggesting methods of recording ocular signs. A diagnosis sheet for any ophthalmic examination is given in Figure 1.1 and may be

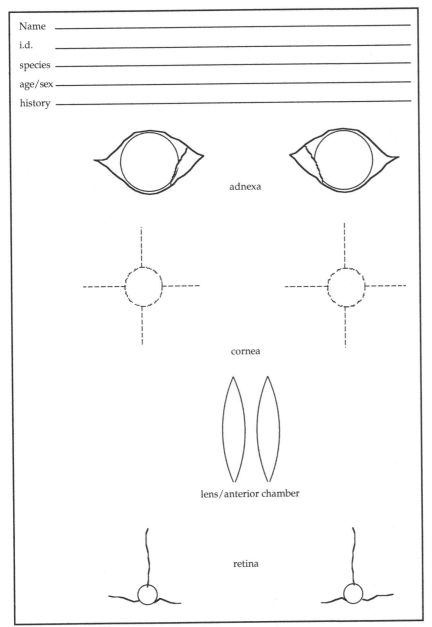

Figure 1.1 An example of a diagnostic sheet for ophthalmic examination. Note that a full-page version of this figure (available for photocopying and use by readers) is provided on page 95

copied to give an acceptable method of recording ophthalmic lesions in an emergency (see page 95). Alternatively, readers can devise their own scheme to record ophthalmic signs in an emergency situation and in everyday practice.

1.3 Equipment and aids required to deal with the ocular emergency

It has already been indicated that a simple tonometer is required as a basic tool in every practice. What other items should be close to hand to deal with the ocular emergency? Clearly a good ophthalmoscope is essential. Although many veterinary ophthalmologists arm themselves with an indirect ophthalmoscope and slit lamp as basic tools for an ophthalmic examination, in reality a good direct ophthalmoscope will suffice in a general practice setting. As well as enabling examination of the retina at the 0 D setting and the iris and lens at a setting of +10 D, the direct ophthalmoscope is a very useful magnifying lens for the cornea and adnexa when used at +20 D. With a powerful halogen light source such an instrument, although not looking as impressive as a slit lamp, is much less expensive and yet invaluable if used to maximum effect.

A cheap solution for indirect ophthalmoscopy is a plastic 20 D lens held close to the cornea of the animal and a simple pen torch held to the ear of the examiner (Figure 1.2a). This will enable the examiner to view most of the fundus at one time. For examination of the iridocorneal angle a goniolens might be considered worth obtaining, the Koeppe or Franklin lenses being particularly easy to use (Figure 1.2b). Their application is considered further in Appendix A.

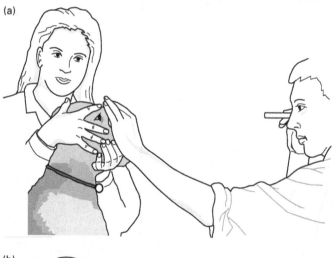

(a)

(b)

Figure 1.2 Indirect ophthalmoscopy using a plastic 20 D lens held close to the cornea of the animal and a simple pen torch held to the ear of the examiner. (a) Uni-ocular indirect ophthalmoscopy; (b) binocular indirect ophthalmoscopy

Schirmer tear test strips are valuable and should be used to determine tear production or lack of it before any manipulation of the eye is attempted. The dyes fluorescein and rose bengal should be a key part of the diagnostic armamentarium: their use is described further in the corneal section. Bacteriology swabs should be at hand as should a Kimura spatula for the collection of cytology samples. Kimura spatulas are expensive and the blunt end of a Bard-Parker scalpel handle may be used in its place. A more recent innovation is that of cytology brushes (Figure 1.3) which increase cell recovery and reduce sampling-induced damage to recovered cells (Wills et al. 1997).

Local anaesthetic is necessary in many instances. Profound anaesthesia can be obtained by soaking a cotton-tipped applicator and pressing it firmly onto an area of conjunctiva before, for instance, the collection of a conjunctival biopsy in the conscious patient.

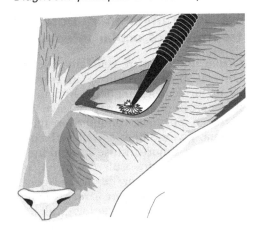

Figure 1.3 Use of a cytology brush will increase cell recovery and lessen sampling-induced damage to recovered cells

Figures 1.4 to 1.7 show both the basic, as well as the more specialized, sets of ophthalmic equipment.

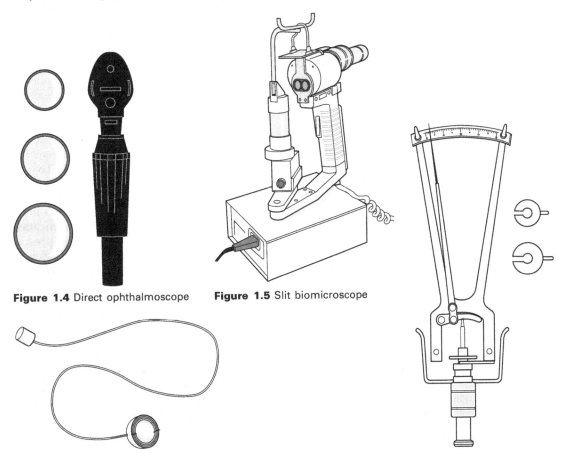

Figure 1.4 Direct ophthalmoscope   **Figure 1.5** Slit biomicroscope

Figure 1.6 Gonio lens

Figure 1.7 Schiotz tonometer

1.4 Some preliminary notes on treatment of ocular infections

Ocular infections are generally considered as adnexal diseases resulting in conjunctivitis, be it purulent, chemotic or hyperaemic. But infection of the eye may involve the orbit, giving a purulent cellulitis; or the corneal stroma, giving either a well-defined stromal abscess or a more diffuse stromal infiltration; or may be intra-ocular, with a purulent anterior uveitis or a more generalized panophthalmitis. There are several differences between the bacteriological investigation of an ocular infection and an infection involving skin or soft tissue. The most important difference is the frequent paucity of organisms isolated from the eye. This means that when a swab from the conjunctiva is taken into transport medium and later plated onto agar, there is often only a scanty growth of organisms. Plating directly from the swab is much to be preferred. The prevalence of fungal disease of the ocular surface, especially in warm climates, means that a Saboraud's agar plate should be used as well as a blood agar plate. This, in practice, mostly applies to equine ocular infection and to cases in other species where the trauma has been caused by vegetable matter such as a thorn or a branch.

Antibiotic sensitivities for cultured organisms should be viewed with caution: sensitivities are based on likely blood levels of orally or parenterally delivered antibiotics, and the much higher concentrations are given locally by topically applied antibiotics. Whenever possible MIC-determinations will be of greater value than sensitivity testing based on disc diffusion.

There are many instances of drug resistance in bacteria affecting the ocular surface, especially with regard to gentamicin in the treatment of *Pseudomonas*. The use of fortified preparations, as detailed in Appendix C, has been widespread to overcome this problem of resistance but itself is likely to induce resistance at higher levels. The more appropriate alternative would be any of the less commonly used aminoglycosides, such as tobramycin, to which resistance has been less frequently noted. More potent antibiotics include the quinolones: ofloxacin, ciprofloxacin or norfloxacin. Their mode of action, inhibiting DNA gyrase, is novel and

thus resistance to other drugs would not affect these drugs. As with every antibiotic, however, the important factors in discouraging resistance are regular dosing and persistence with treatment until well after the signs have gone. Inadequate dose frequency and cessation of treatment while there are still some organisms present are likely to lead to resistance development.

Apart from such considerations, we recommend two drugs for general topical use in external eye disease in dogs and cats respectively before bacteriology results are available. These are fusidic acid for dogs and chlortetracycline for cats. These choices are made given the common organisms seen in these species. Normal bacterial conjunctival flora in dogs include *Staphylococci* and *Streptococci* (Gerding and Kakoma 1990). Normal flora in cats include these Gram-positive species; common agents causing disease are more likely to be Gram-negative organisms, *Chlamydia* and *Mycoplasma* (Gerding and Kakoma 1990), more sensitive to the tetracyclines. Better than either of these for transcorneal penetration, and thus indicated in intra-ocular infections, is chloramphenicol. This has a wide range of activity, important when the full identity of the organism involved is not known.

The use of general broad-spectrum antibiotics is based on the assumption that the result of bacteriological culture and sensitivity will not be available for at least two or three days from the time of sampling, even given a courier dispatch service and the most rapid laboratory turn-around. Clearly a more rapid system is needed to give an indication of which class of infectious agent is present and whether corneal integrity is threatened. In an emergency situation it is important to be proficient in preparing bacteriological stains of smeared swab samples or scrapes from cornea or conjunctiva. Three such smears, stained with Gram's stain, Diff Quik (Giemsa) and lactophenol cotton blue will allow a very rapid assessment of whether a Gram-positive organism is present, probably sensitive to fusidic acid, a Gram-negative organism requiring chloramphenicol or tetracycline, or a fungal agent best treated with ketaconazole. It may be argued that in not every case is the offending organism seen on a scrape or smear – exfoliative cytology in

Box 1.2 Ocular pain

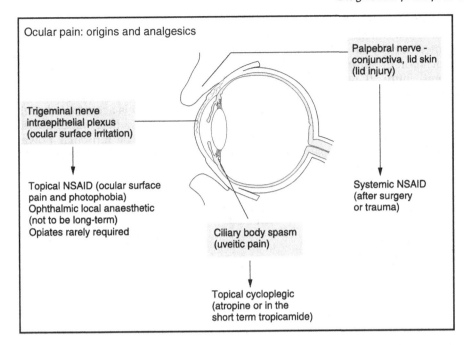

Ocular pain: origins and analgesics

Palpebral nerve - conjunctiva, lid skin (lid injury)

Trigeminal nerve intraepithelial plexus (ocular surface irritation)

Topical NSAID (ocular surface pain and photophobia) Ophthalmic local anaesthetic (not to be long-term) Opiates rarely required

Systemic NSAID (after surgery or trauma)

Ciliary body spasm (uveitic pain)

Topical cycloplegic (atropine or in the short term tropicamide)

such cases will render a neutrophilic infiltrate, which even if no organisms are seen should be taken as evidence of bacterial infection (Lavach et al. 1977, Severin and Thrall 1981, Ugomori et al. 1991).

1.5 Analgesia in ocular emergencies

All too often in veterinary medicine, these authors feel, we pay too little attention to pain relief either post-operatively or after a traumatic incident. The fact that many animals appear to cope stoically with what we would consider an acutely painful injury or condition should not let us negate our duty to provide adequate, or perhaps it should be said better than adequate, pain relief. The eye is an exquisitely delicate organ with an ample nociceptive nervous supply. This is especially so on the ocular surface, with a nerve network at a very superficial level in the cornea. The ophthalmic division of the trigeminal nerve innervates the cornea through the long ciliary nerves, radiating into the stroma from the limbus, there losing their myelin sheaths and forming a subepithelial plexus (Prince et al. 1960). From there fine axons, devoid even of Schwann cells, pierce the epithelium forming

an intra-epithelial plexus highly sensitive to pain and to changes in temperature. These bare nerve endings are therefore less than 50 µm from the ocular surface. This detail of anatomy is highlighted to impress upon the reader the importance of analgesia in ocular surface disease (see Figure 1.8, Spreull 1966).

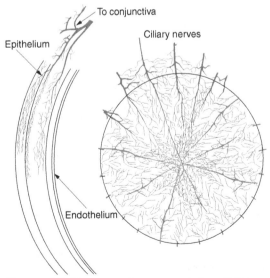

To conjunctiva

Ciliary nerves

Epithelium

Endothelium

Figure 1.8 Diagrammatic representation of the sensory nerve pattern of the cornea (after Prince et al. 1960)

In the emergency setting such analgesia may involve topical local anaesthetic such as amethocaine or proxymethocaine, but this can only be used in the short term because of toxic effects on corneal epithelium (Grant and Acosta 1994). Such local analgesia may be required fully to examine the eye. The use of profound sedatives such as the alpha 2 agonists alone perhaps should be questioned, since while they render the animal more easily handled, the degree of analgesia may be insufficient. Parenterally administered analgesics such as a non-steroidal anti-inflammatory agent (e.g. carprofen or flunixine meglumine) or in more severe circumstances an opiate such as methadone or butorphenol should be considered in such cases and for more medium-term pain relief. In the cat ketoprofen should be used in the place of carprofen.

In the case of pain associated with profound miosis, as seen in uveitis, the main cause of pain is spasm of the cilary body. For this reason a mydriastic cycloplegic (ciliary-body paralysing agent) such as atropine may be a better analgesic than a standard non-steroidal or even opiate analgesic. While tropicamide is more rapidly acting it has less cycloplegic action than atropine, so it is the latter drug which should be used as a ciliary-body spasmolytic agent in uveitis.

1.6 Dealing with ocular emergencies in horses and ruminants

Ophthalmology is a wonderfully trans-species discipline. While at first it was intended that this book would aim solely at small animal veterinarians, the authors then decided that including horses and food animals would be appropriate. We still focus on the small animal but include large animals, and particularly companion equine ophthalmic emergencies throughout the text. There are some significant differences in these species, particularly considering the approaches both to clinical examination and to medication, and it is these which are covered by this section.

1.6.1 Techniques facilitating large animal ocular examination

Examination in a light environment renders ophthalmoscopy difficult and thus a darkened box should be sought or, if this is not possible, a large sheet of fabric (preferably dark blue or black) can be put over the head of the examiner as well as of the horse, as a tent to simulate a darkened room.

The examination of a painful eye is always somewhat tricky, but this is accentuated with horses and food animals where the temperament of the animal and the muscular power of the blepharospastic eyelids combine to

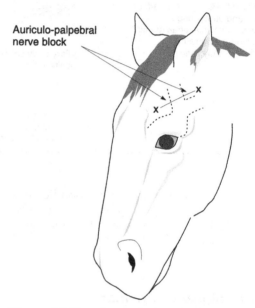

Figure 1.9 Use of an auriculo palpebral nerve block in the horse

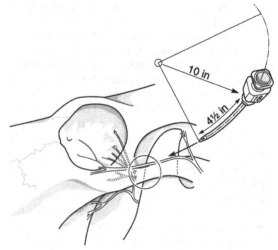

Figure 1.10 Needle placement for a Petersen block in cattle (after Lavach, 1990)

render safe visualization of the ocular surface difficult. Mild sedation remedies the first problem, but may not ameliorate the covering of the globe by lids in muscular spasm. The use of an auriculopalpebral nerve block in the horse (Figure 1.9) and the Petersen block, commonly used in cattle (Figure 1.10), allow full examination without the interference of eyelid spasm (Lavach 1990). Retrobulbar muscle spasm may give considerable enophthalmos in cattle which, again, complicates examination. Here the Petersen block ameliorates the problem (Lavach 1990).

1.6.2 Techniques facilitating large animal ocular therapeutics

Here we consider three techniques – first the simple method of subconjunctival drug delivery. This is particularly useful in ruminant diseases such as New Forest Eye – infectious bovine keratoconjunctivitis (IBK) associated with *Moraxella bovis* and *Mycoplasma bovicula*. In the treatment of IBK, systemic tetracycline therapy may be necessary (Lavach 1990); but often a subconjunctival depot injection of an appropriate antibiotic such as cloxacillin is efficacious for around three days before requiring a second application.

There are some theoretical considerations to take note of before accepting that this is the optimum route for all large animal ocular medication. Drugs injected subconjunctivally might be supposed to enter the eye by transscleral penetration. A significant volume of injected solutions, however, has been shown in other species to exit from the injection site and be absorbed by topical transcorneal penetration. Entry by the trans-scleral route can be optimized by a deeper injection at a sub-Tenon's level. This can be important when the aim is to give high intra-ocular levels of antibiotic rather than corneal or ocular surface medication. Such injections may require considerable sedation: in any case subconjunctival injections should be attempted only after topical ocular surface anaesthesia.

The main indication for subconjunctival delivery in the horse or small animal is the injection of antibiotics for the emergency management of anterior segment infection. Corticosteroid depot injections can also be given in this manner for treatment of corneal inflammation. In either case, subconjunctival medication supplements topical therapy rather than replacing it. Similarly the application of mydriatics in emergency situations by the subconjunctival route might be considered in equine or in small animal anterior uveitis. There are, however, potential problems of systemic absorption of potent autonomic agents with the injection of drugs such as atropine and adrenaline.

The need to provide frequent topical ocular medication to painful eyes is especially important in equine uveitis and ulcerative keratitis. In these conditions horses will often vigorously resent regular instillation of medication and thus placement of a drug delivery system allowing interference with the eye to be minimized is advantageous. Two systems have been reported. The nasolacrimal lavage system involves a length of tubing placed from the nasal nasolacrimal punctum to reach the upper end of the duct (Figure 1.11). Drug solutions can then be instilled topically up the nasolacrimal duct. While having the considerable advantage of

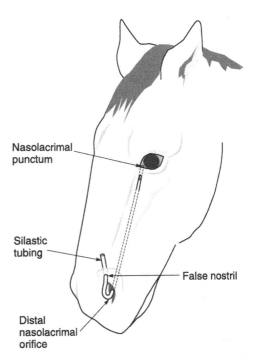

Nasolacrimal punctum

Silastic tubing

False nostril

Distal nasolacrimal orifice

Figure 1.11 Length of tubing is placed from the nasal nasolacrimal punctum to reach the upper end of the duct

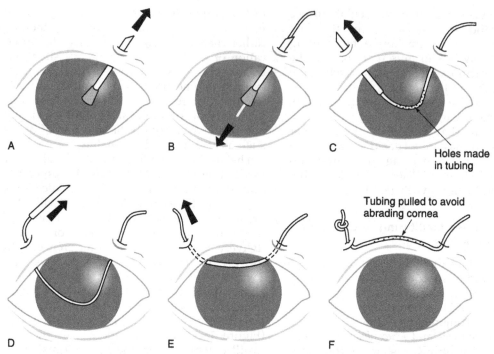

A   B   C

Holes made
in tubing

Tubing pulled to avoid
abrading cornea

D   E   F

Figure 1.12 Transpalpebral drug delivery via insertion of a cannula. (A) The cannula is placed through the lid from the conjunctival to the dermal surface; (B) the tubing is drawn through the cannula from the dermal to the conjunctival surface and the cannula withdrawn; (C) the cannula is placed through the lid from the conjunctival to the dermal surface, ensuring that the tubing has been removed; (D) the tubing is drawn through the cannula and then the cannula is withdrawn over the tubing; (E) the tubing is placed well above the globe surface; (F) the tubing is secured by knotting

ease of placement this system has the disadvantage that drug delivery may also flush potentially infectious material from the nasolacrimal duct back to the ocular surface.

In many cases the preferable technique is one of transpalpebral drug delivery, as illustrated diagrammatically (Figure 1.12A–F). The optimal technique is a through-and-through placement with the tube anchored by a knot on the dermal (external) surface of the lid. This is preferable to the technique using a single lid passage flare-ended tube: the flared end causes at best ocular irritation and at worst corneal damage. Securing the tubing after a second passage through the lid may be more time consuming to perform but avoids any possibility of corneal damage. Polyethylene tubing (PE 190) or a premature infant nasogastric feeding tube is used, with holes cut at the appropriate site to allow the drug solution to bathe the ocular surface. Horses, and especially those in considerable ocular discomfort, need profound sedation before

the placement is attempted. Local anaesthesia with intradermal lignocaine and topical administration of proparacaine or proxymetacaine should also be given.

Two key features of tube placement should be noted. First, the guide used to penetrate the lid, either a 14 gauge needle or preferably a 10 gauge flexible angiocatheter, always passes from the conjunctival (internal) to the dermal (external) side of the lid. In this way the cornea is always protected from abrasion or penetration. This does necessitate removal of the hub of the needle or catheter for the second pass through the lid, ensuring that the guide can be passed through the lid over the tubing after placement through the lid.

The second feature to note is that the tubing should be placed as deep in the conjunctival fornix as possible, to ensure that corneal abrasion does not occur while the delivery system is in place. Then a small quantity of drug is injected into the tubing, followed by a considerable bolus of air to force the solution through the delivery system to the ocular surface. The alternative is to use a constant infusion device to deliver a constant small flow to the ocular surface: such equipment can readily be fastened to the head-collar, as can injection ports if frequent bolus deliveries are given.

A spray medication can be a valuable means of delivering drugs to the anterior surface of the equine eye. The usual eye medication is transferred to a spray unit and the drizzle on the cornea is likely to cause less reflex tearing; also the horse is less affected by the spray than by topical delivery from traditional drop-bottles and eye-medication applied at the lateral canthus with a 1 ml syringe.

When using topical antibiotics in the horse, one must always consider the possibility of fungal overgrowth. Thus if the infection is not responding to topical medication, perform a corneal scraping and investigate for fungus by microscopy as well as culture. For an example of broad-spectrum antibiotic solutions for equine keratitis see Appendix C.

1.7 Ocular emergencies in exotic species

The majority of ocular emergencies in small mammals, birds, reptiles and amphibia can be dealt with by simple extrapolation from what is known from dealing with the dog and cat: a corneal ulcer in a parrot can be treated in much the same way as in a dog. On the other hand there are some significant differences which should be taken into consideration when dealing with an emergency in these species. These are discussed throughout the text but are gathered in Table 1.1 for ease of reference.

Table 1.1 Where ocular emergencies in exotic animals differ from the dog and cat

Adnexal masses in lower vertebrates	Often not neoplastic but inflammatory
Uveitis in lower vertebrates	Often associated with Gram-negative septicaemia
Uveitis in lower vertebrates and birds	Miosis requires non-depolarizing muscle relaxant, not atropine
Traumatic keratitis in parrots	Reported particularly in Amazons and mynnah birds and requiring supportive therapy predominantly with artificial tears
Pox virus in parrots	Early serious discharge becomes mucopurulent but the main lesions are lid scabs from self-trauma – prevent this with supportive tear replacement or bathing with mild baby shampoo
Dacryocystitis in rabbits	Causing significant white purulent ocular discharge – requires nasolacrimal cannulation and systemic antibiosis with enrofloxacin often the best therapeutic agent
Myxomatosis in rabbits	Swollen lids and white mucopurulent discharge or, in vaccinated animals, adnexal masses and lid distortion
Uveitis in rabbits	May be associated with Pasteurella infection or encephalitozoan cuniculi-related phacoclastic uveitis

Chapter 2

Commonly presented conditions – a problem-oriented approach

2.1 The red eye

This ophthalmic term refers to an eye in which the white of the eye is abnormally reddened. There are other conditions resulting in redness of the eye, such as hyphaema in which the blood in the anterior chamber imparts a red coloration to the eye. In addition trauma may lead to subconjunctival haemorrhage giving a red eye. Here, however, we will confine discussion to eyes reddened in a more diffuse manner. The four classic differential diagnoses of the red eye thus defined are

- Conjunctivitis
- Uveitis
- Glaucoma
- Scleritis/episcleritis complex (less common).

One key point to note when considering the differential diagnosis of this clinical sign is that the 'white of the eye' is made up anatomically of three structures: the conjunctiva, the episclera and the sclera, each with its own perilimbal vascular plexus. Inflammation of each layer of the covering of the eye results in vascular engorgement in the corresponding plexus. These can be differentiated to a degree by careful examination but also pharmacologically. On examination, the conjunctival vascular plexus moves as the conjunctiva is gently moved while the deeper plexuses cannot be moved to this degree. Differentiating between episcleral and scleral

plexus involvement, however, calls for the application of the topical vasoconstrictor phenylephrine (see Appendix C). This will constrict and thus visually obliterate an episcleral plexus engorged through inflammatory involvement but does not have the same effect on the deeper scleral plexus.

A second key point in the differentiation of the red eye is that redness can include a number of different clinical presentations. The redness may be a diffuse feature or one associated either with numerous small blood vessels or a few engorged vessels. Each of these different rednesses can be associated with a different diagnosis. A mild overall redness normally indicates conjunctivitis, while a deeper more 'angry' red close to the limbus is typical of ciliary flush, often associated with uveitis. Deeply engorged episcleral vessels against a generally white scleral background more often indicates glaucoma.

The most important feature to note in coming to a diagnosis does not, however, concern the redness itself but rather other signs in the eye. The eye with conjunctivitis is often in other respects unremarkable. A causative feature may be an eyelid abnormality such as entropion, ectopic cilium or distichiasis. An associated ocular sign in lymphocytic/plasmacytic conjunctivitis may be corneal involvement with chronic superficial keratitis (pannus). Similarly, the bulbar surface of the nictitating membrane may be involved in follicular conjunctivitis (plasmoma) and indeed the

Table 2.1 Differential diagnosis of the red eye

Feature	Acute conjunctivitis	Acute uveitis	Acute glaucoma
Pain	Painfree to mild irritation	Mild to severe pain	Can be extremely severe
Vision	Unaffected except in systemic disease such as distemper where the blindness is central rather than ocular	Slight impairment with miosis through to blindness caused by retinal detachment	Often severe impairment to profound blindness
Discharge	Moderate to copious and may be serous, mucoid or purulent	Generally confined to lacrimation because of painful and increased blinking	Generally confined to lacrimation because of pain and increased blinking
Blood vessels	Conjunctival hyperaemia with mobile vessels often associated with oedematous inflamed conjunctiva. Note that lid and globe conjunctivae are both affected	Limbal flush and diffuse redness in episcleral vessels deeper than those of the conjunctiva. Note that the bulbar vessels are involved while those of the lid are normal	Episcleral vessel engorgement and congestion with stasis hyperaemia
Cornea	Clear unless keratitis is also occurring	Varying from clear through being affected with keratic precipitates to being frankly oedematous	A classically steamy or ground-glass diffuse corneal oedema
Aqueous	Clear	Affected with cells and fibrin giving flare, hypopyon or hyphaema	Clear
Iris	Unaffected	Muddy, thickened or dark with indistinct surface features and often iridolenticular adhesions (synechiae)	Usually of normal appearance but possibly a shallow anterior chamber
Pupil	Unaffected	Small (miotic) irregular or fixed with a sluggish response to light	Dilated and fixed
Intraocular pressure	Unaffected	Decreased because of ciliary body involvement	Increased
Lens	Unaffected	May be involved with pigment deposition or synechiae	May be in situ, subluxated or luxated secondary to globe enlargement in buphthalmos
Posterior segment	Unaffected except in systemic diseases such as distemper	Hyalitis, pars planitis, chorioretinitis or optic neuritis may occur in panuveitis	Often not visible but retinal vascular attenuation or optic nerve cupping may occur

Differential diagnosis of the red eye

- Conjunctivitis Note involvement of palpebral and bulbar conjunctiva
- Uveitis Note generalized globe redness often increasing at limbus (ciliary flush); note other ocular signs – keratic precipitates, hypopyon, miosis, posterior synechiae, also pain and photophobia in acute cases
- Glaucoma Congestion/injection of episcleral vessels; other ocular signs – blindness, pain
- Episcleritis or scleritis Deeper vascular involvement with swelling at appropriate level

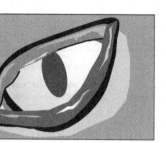

(a)

Conjunctivitis

Redness of lid and globe conjunctiva

Diffuse redness

Conjunctival swelling (chemosis)

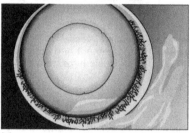

(b)

Uveitis

Intense redness, increasing near limbus (ciliary flush)

Little or no lid redness

Note other signs of miosis, intravascular inflammatory deposits (hypopyon or keratic precipates)

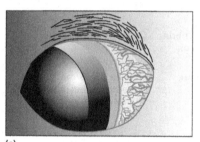

(c)

Classic acute glaucoma

Individual engorged vessels

Little redness in between here with lens luxation

Note other signs of visual disturbance, pain, optic disc cupping, lens luxation (as here)

Figure 2.1 Form and appearance of redness

roughened inner surface of the nictitating membrane in these circumstances may itself be a focus of irritation.

The most important differentials for a red eye involve other marked ocular signs concurrent with the redness. The eye with uveitis exhibits miosis, flare, keratic precipitates or hypopyon with posterior synechiae as a critical sequel to pupillary margin inflammation. The uveitic eye is often painful and photophobic, while the glaucomatous eye is equally if not more painful but less often photophobic. The glaucomatous eye may have Haab's striae (fractures of Descemet's membrane appearing as white lines across the cornea) or frank corneal oedema manifesting as a ground-glass appearance of the grey to white cornea. The eye with sudden onset glaucoma is often blind, while the uveitic eye is rarely blind unless sight is obscured by gross flare, hypopyon or intense miosis.

One unusual and generally benign cause of the red eye is Horner's syndrome (Figure 2.2). The redness of the conjunctiva of the third eyelid protruded in this syndrome is often mistaken for a unilateral red eye. Close examination of the eye shows the other signs of Horner's syndrome – a miotic pupil and ptosis (drooping) of the upper eyelid. Use of topical 1% phenylephrine ameliorates these signs. It also shows that the correct diagnosis has been reached and defines the position of the damage to the ocular sympathetic nerve supply by the time taken for the administration to have its effect. A rapid amelioration indicates that denervation hypersensitivity of sympathetically innervated structures has occurred with a third order neuropathy. Further details of the diagnosis and prognosis of Horner's syndrome can be found in Neer's (1984) excellent review of the subject.

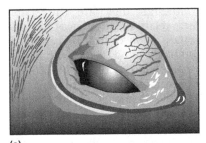

(a)

Episcleritis and scleritis

Nodular or diffuse with or without corneal involvement

Deeper vascular engorgement pales less with topical phenylephrine

Figure 2.2 Other causes of ocular redness

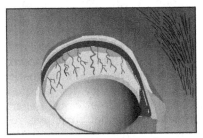

(b)

Vessel engorgement through vascular compromise

No other ocular signs

Diagnosis on colour flow Doppler ultrasound

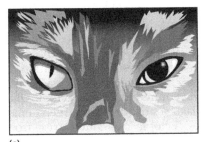

(c)

Raised apparently reddened third eyelid

Possible Horner's syndrome

Possible ocular pain with globe retraction

2.2 The painful eye

The spectrum of what we might call ocular irritation ranges from the mild but chronic discomfort caused by an ectopic cilium to the rapid onset severe pain of acute glaucoma. Here we will consider first the acutely painful eye, since these are the emergency situations, before discussing briefly conditions with chronic ocular discomfort. To some extent there is an overlap in presentation in the middle of the nociceptive spectrum.

The acutely painful eye may be the result of a traumatic episode with tissue disruption by external injury, or of two conditions in which ocular damage is the result of internal injurious mechanisms: uveitis and glaucoma. Diagnosis of these latter two conditions relies on evaluation of ocular signs on ophthalmoscopy. Their differential diagnosis presented above.

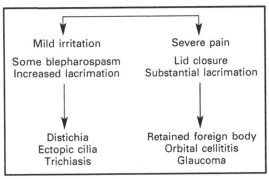

Mild irritation

Some blepharospasm
Increased lacrimation

Severe pain

Lid closure
Substantial lacrimation

Distichia
Ectopic cilia
Trichiasis

Retained foreign body
Orbital cellititis
Glaucoma

Box 2.1 Ocular pain

Understanding the origin of the pain is important for its relief. If it stems from ciliary muscle spasm, as in uveitis, then paralysis of this muscle will reduce pain. If it stems from a defective tear film exposing corneal nerve endings to drying effects then tear replacement is required. However, the origin of pain in ocular disease is not in all cases completely understood. Where does the photophobia in uveitis originate, especially as it can be ameliorated by the use of topical non-steroidal anti-inflammatories in many cases? And where does the acute pain in glaucoma originate and why do rabbits not seem to be at all concerned by it? There are as many questions left to answer in ophthalmology as there are satisfactorily solved!

Ocular trauma can result in external and/or internal tissue disruption and widely differing degrees of pain. The pain accompanying corneal injury can too easily be underestimated (although anyone wearing contact lenses knows the quite severe pain of an apparently minor ocular surface abrasion). There seems to be quite a range of response to corneal ulceration between individual animals: some with a deep ulcer will appear to feel little discomfort while others with only a mild surface abrasion will exhibit marked blepharospasm and lacrimation suggesting a considerable nociceptive response. The anatomy and physiology of corneal nociception is discussed below The reason for this difference in response may possibly be individual variation in degree of corneal innervation between animals; or more likely differences in individual tolerance of painful stimuli; or conceivably because superficial ocular surface damage massively stimulates trigeminal pain receptors while deeper stromal injury actually exposes fewer pain-fibre endings.

The same variation can be seen in glaucoma. Some animals with early rises in ocular pressure have exceptionally painful eyes while others with catastrophic rises in pressure accompanied by buphthalmos seem not to suffer pain although they are irreversibly blind. This may relate to differences in intra-ocular innervation or in central perception of pain but is also likely to be linked with degeneration of pain fibres once intra-ocular pressure has been high for some time.

The differential diagnosis of less severe ocular discomfort centres mostly around causes of physical irritation (see Box 2.1). Ocular foreign bodies are an obvious potential cause of irritation which may be mild or severe. These may be readily visible but often are hidden from immediate view in the conjunctival fornix or behind the nictitating membrane. Local anaesthesia with topical amethocaine drops (or other local anaesthetics: see Appendix C) is necessary for adequate investigation while in some cases general anaesthesia may be essential. Irritative foci may be integral to ocular structures rather than from an external agency such as a foreign body. Ectopic cilia, distichial lashes or hair from surrounding skin (trichiasis) may be responsible for considerable ocular irritation. Investigation of these lashes again often requires local anaesthesia. Magnification is often necessary to diagnose distichiasis and almost always required to localize ectopic cilia.

Distichial lashes arise from the meibomian gland orifices. Ectopic cilia often arise from meibomian glands but through the conjunctiva, or have distinct hair follicles which may occur at any point in the palpebral tissue. This difference is reflected in the treatment techniques for these cilia. Distichia may simply be plucked with forceps. In some cases owners are happy to perform this from time to time. While this may seem optimal to some clients, distichia plucked may recur rapidly. Because new distichia can be shorter and more irritant sometimes such plucking can increase, rather than eliminate, irritation. Distichia can be removed by electrolysis, by cryosurgical ablation or by sharp knife surgery (Lawson 1973, Chambers and Slatter 1984, Wolfley 1987). Electrolysis aims to deal lash by lash with the distichia while cryosurgery on the lids seeks to destroy the meibomian glands from which the lashes originate. Both of these techniques can cause considerable palpebral inflammation and presurgical medication with non-steroidal anti-inflammatory agents is advised. Some veterinary ophthalmologists apply a cold/ice pack to the eyelids after cryosurgery has been performed and leave the pack until the animal wakes up. Sharp-knife surgery aims to remove the meibomian gland seats of the lashes and thus avoids incisions in the lid. In the past lid margin resection was advocated to remove distichia, but the risk of lid scarring is too great to warrant use of that technique today.

Treatment of ectopic cilia requires sharp-knife resection of the area from which the cilia arise. Ectopic cilia often originate together and during surgery a number of hairs may be found together in the thickening on the palpebral conjunctiva.

2.3 The white eye

Normally the term white eye is used to differentiate a quiet or disease-free eye from a red eye, as discussed above, but here we use the term to denote a pathological white appearance. The key here is determination of where the white opacity is within the eye. A white cornea or an opaque aqueous humour prevent visualization of intra-ocular structures beneath it, while iris detail can still be seen around a white lens opacity. The differentiation of an opaque cornea or aqueous is more difficult. A slit beam allows the anterior and posterior faces of the cornea to be identified in the latter case while showing the opacity to be intracorneal in the former. In any case corneal opacification is far more common than is a white aqueous.

A white opacity in front of the lens can only be one of four things

- Cellular invasion
- Oedema
- Scar tissue
- Lipid

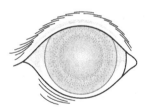

Corneal oedema :
    Glaucoma – note vessel engorgement
    and visual disturbance
    Endothelial dystrophy – diffuse corneal
    opacity often the only sign

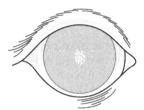

Lipid deposition :
    Lipid dystrophy – central crystalline
    deposition

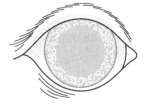

Arcus lipoides cornae – at the limbus :
    associated with hypothyroid or
    lipid metabolic abnormality

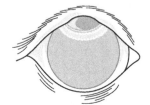

Lipid keratopathy :
    associated with corneal
    vascularization or limbal mass

Figure 2.3 The white eye

All four can occur in the cornea while in the aqueous humour only cellular infiltration and lipid involvement are seen (Figure 2.3). Corneal oedema is a sign of what one might consider a true emergency situation, glaucoma. Other white corneal changes occur mostly in chronic lesions which cannot be considered to be emergencies. Cellular infiltration of the cornea is normally accompanied by vascular invasion, giving a pink hue as seen in chronic superficial keratitis. Corneal oedema, however, gives a classical ground glass appearance through which, when mild, some intra-ocular detail can be seen using a bright light source such as a Finhoff transilluminator. The differential diagnosis of conditions associated with corneal oedema includes

- Glaucoma
- Endothelial dystrophy
- Endothelitis associated with uveitis often after canine adenovirus infection
- Endothelial trauma

The appearance of corneal lipid deposition depends on the type of lipid or lipoprotein involved. Cholesterol, for instance, forms characteristic crystals while low density lipoprotein gives a finer lipid infiltrate. Scar tissue is readily recognizable as such, having a heterogeneous white-grey appearance. Blood vessels are often seen in association with corneal scar tissue.

Cellular infiltration of the aqueous produces a flare which can properly be appreciated only by making use of the Tyndall effect, and thus is not a truly white eye (Figure 2.4). Oedema and scar tissue do not occur in the aqueous, leaving lipid and fibrin deposition as the only reasons for a dense white aqueous humour. Lipid-laden aqueous does indeed give a completely white eye as a very startling diagnostic feature. This could be considered an emergency, given that it disturbs vision and because it can follow uveitis where an abnormally high circulating lipid also occurs. Fibrin in the anterior chamber gives a grey or yellow colour to the aqueous rather than white but signals an emergency in some cases, as it is associated with uveitis. In the vitreous a total retinal detachment could be confused with a white eye, and a posterior chamber tumour may produce a white pupil or leucocoria.

With regard to the lens, cataract is clearly a significant cause of white opacity, but the only cataractous change which could be classed as an emergency is the diabetic cataract. This is an emergency both because it can occur rapidly and be a cause for sudden change in the appearance of the ocular media and visual deterioration, and also because it is a manifestation of a serious systemic endocrine disease.

2.4 The suddenly blind eye

The suddenly blind eye is clearly an emergency first because visual compromise is a cause for concern even if only temporary. Secondly, sudden blindness is often the prelude to permanent blindness.

Sudden blindness is caused through one of four mechanisms.

1. The first mechanism is opacification of the ocular media. The only two conditions in which media opacification occurs with rapid onset are lipid-laden aqueous and diabetic cataract (as covered above under the white eye) or vitreal or retinal haemorrhage.
2. The second mechanism is disruption of retinal function. Rapid deterioration in

---

Differential diagnosis of the blue/white eye

- Where is the opacity? – cornea, aqueous, lens?
- What is the appearance of the opacity? – dense crystalline, ground glass, etc.?
- How widespread is the opacity? – across whole cornea, focal, only in pupil?

- Cornea   Corneal lipidosis (dense white, diffuse or micro crystalline)
                 Corneal scar (diffuse, often off-white striate appearance)
- Aqueous   Lipid-laden aqueous (diffuse throughout aqueous)
                 Hypopyon (ventrally often with a horizontal margin dorsally)
- Lens   Cataract (only seen within pupil, behind lens)

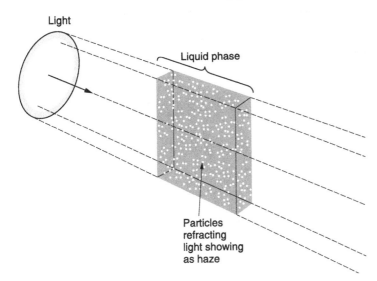

Light

Liquid phase

Particles
refracting
light showing
as haze

Figure 2.4 As happens (or rather, used to happen) in a smoke-filled cinema, the light lens highlights the particles in the gas phase, or in the aqueous the liquid phase. This is the key diagnostic test to evaluate flare in anterior uveitis

retinal activity occurs either as a consequence of complete retinal detachment or failure of retinal electrical function in sudden acquired retinal degeneration. Retinal detachment may occur as the result of posterior uveitis, hypertension or trauma. It may be related to inherited disease such as retinal dysplasia or Collie eye anomaly. The syndrome of sudden acquired retinal degeneration (SARD) gives no observable retinal changes at the time of first visual loss, but electroretinography shows no measurable retinal electrical activity. Later indicators of retinal degeneration such as increased tapetal reflectivity occur, but as these are not present early in the disease they are not helpful diagnostic signs in the emergency situation.

3. The third mechanism for sudden loss of vision is optic nerve dysfunction. Glaucoma and optic neuritis are the two conditions most commonly giving rise to dysfunction although tumours of the optic nerve or surrounding structures can on occasion cause loss of function.

Although we associate glaucoma with ocular disease at the iridocorneal angle the mechanism of visual loss relates to damage at the optic nerve head. Cupping of the optic nerve head is a visible change, but before this happens pressure necrosis of the nerve fibres coursing over the edge of the cribriform plate to enter the optic nerve itself accounts for visual loss.

Optic neuritis may be visible at the papilla by fundoscopy, with a swollen optic nerve head with or without peripapillary haemorrhages. On rare occasions the inflammatory process occurs not at the optic nerve head but in the nerve at the retrobulbar level. Diagnosis of retrobulbar optic neuritis is generally by exclusion but ultrasonographic or magnetic resonance imaging (MRI) or computerized tomography (CT) can show a swollen retrobulbar optic nerve, and electroretinography reveals normal retinal activity.

Tumours of the optic nerve itself, such as optic nerve meningiomas, can cause visual disturbance as can adjacent masses pressing on the optic nerve. Of these pituitary tumours are classical causes of bilateral visual disturbance through pressure on the optic chiasm. Such cases highlight the necessity for a full clinical work up. They manifest also in endocrine abnormalities such as diabetes insipidus, and diagnosis can be aided by tests such as the ACTH stimulation test.

4. The fourth mechanism causing sudden visual loss is central blindness. Here all parameters of ocular function are normal and the diagnosis rests on electrodiagnosis with abnormalities shown in visually evoked potentials by electroencephalography. Magnetic resonance or CT imaging

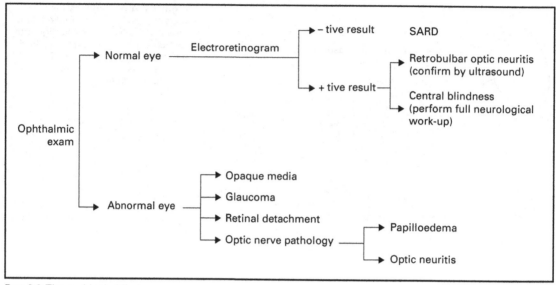

Box 2.2 The suddenly blind eye

Differential diagnosis of the suddenly blind eye

• Opacification of media	Lipid laden aqueous Diabetic cataract Intraocular haemorrhage (aqueous or vitreous)
• Disruption of retinal function	Retinal detachment Sudden Acquired Retinal Degeneration (SARD)

• Optic nerve dysfunction	Optic neuritis
	Glaucomatous optic neuropathy
	Optic nerve compression
	    Meningioma
	    Pituitary tumour at the optic chiasm

• Central blindness	Other intracranial space occupying lesion
	    ? raising intracranial pressure
	    ? causing compression of optic radiation

may reveal an intracranial mass or a diagnosis of generalized disease such as granulomatous meningio-encephalitis may be made. Such a condition may also account for some cases of optic neuritis.

2.5 Ocular lesions in systemic disease

Several of the diseases mentioned above, from diabetic cataract to granulomatous

meningo-encephalitis (GME), are ocular manifestations of a systemic condition (Table 2.2). The prevalence of ocular abnormality as a sign of systemic disease shows the importance of a thorough general work up for all animals presenting with ocular disease. The fact that the ocular signs are the reason for emergency presentation should not detract from a thorough clinical examination of the whole animal as soon as possible. The systemic diseases producing ocular signs are shown in Table 2.3.

Table 2.2 Ocular lesions in systemic disease (provided by T.F. Evans)

Disease	Species	Ocular change	Aetiology
Vitamin A deficiency	Eq, bo, ov	Night blindness, poor PLRs	Less production of rhodopsin
Hyperadrenocorticism	Ca	Corneal ulcers, KCS, hypertensive retinopathy, SARD	Hypercortisolaemia
Infectious bovine rhinotracheitis (IBR)	Bo	Conjunctivitis, blepharaospasm, cornea generally clear	
Diabetes mellitus	Ca, fe	Cataract	Osmotic (sorbitol, glucose and aldose reductase)
Hyperthyroidism	Fe	Retinal detachment, perivascular cuffing, tortuous retinal vessels	Hypertension
Chr/acute renal failure	Ca, fe	Retinal detachment, perivascular cuffing, tortuous retinal vessels	Hypertension
Toxoplasmosis	Fe, ca	Anterior uveitis, chorioretinitis	*Toxoplasma gondi* tachyzoites
Canine distemper	Ca, ferret	Conjunctivitis, KCS, chorioretinitis, brown retinal scars	Canine distemper virus
Feline herpes virus	Fe	Conjunctivitis, chemosis, dentritic keratitis	Feline herpes virus 1
Chlamydiosis	Fe, avian	Conjunctivitis, chemosis	*Chlamydia psittaci*
Equine viral arteritis	Eq	Corneal opacity, uveitis, conjunctivitis	EVA-virus
Equine herpes virus	Eq	Conjunctivitis, dendritic keratitis	EHV-1
Feline infectious peritonitis	Fe	Uveitis	Feline coronavirus
Leptospirosis	Eq	Anterior uveitis, equine recurrent uveitis, secondary cataracts	*Leptospira interrogans*
Thiamine deficiency	Fe, eq, bo, ov	Blindness, ataxia	
Listeriosis	Bo, ov, su	Chorioretinitis, blindness (unilateral or bilateral), KCS	*Listeria monocytogenes* bacteraemia
Bovine virus diarrhoea (BVD)	Bo	Cataract, vitreal opacities, optic nerve atrophy, retinal dysplasia	
Liver disease	Ca, fe, eq	Scleral icterus	Hyperbilirubinaemia
Lymphosarcoma	Ca, fe	Uveitis, retinal haemorrhages, secondary glaucoma	Neoplasia, metastasis, phagocytosis
GME	Ca		
Erlichiosis	Ca	Uveitis, retinal haemorrhages, optic neuritis	*Ehrlichia canis*
Taurine deficiency	Fe	Central retinal atrophy (hyperreflectivity in area centralis)	

References are available in Gelatt (1999) and Lavach (1990).

Table 2.3 Systemic diseases with ocular associations having emergency implications

Canine distemper	Conjunctivitis
	Keratoconjunctivitis sicca
	Chorioretinitis
Canine adenoviral hepatitis	Corneal oedema – 'blue eye'
	Anterior uveitis – endothelitis
Feline dysautonomia	Dilated unresponsive pupils
Feline herpes virus	Conjunctivitis, keratoconjunctivitis
	Corneal ulceration
Feline chlamydial infection	Conjunctivitis, chemosis
Feline FIV infection	Uveitis
Feline FIP infection	Anterior uveitis
Feline Felv infection	Anterior uveitis, uveal lymphosarcoma
Feline chlamydial infection	Conjunctivitis, chemosis
Rickettsial infections	Anterior uveitis
Bacterial toxaemia	Anterior uveitis
	Chorioretinitis
Rickettsial and fungal disease	Anterior uveitis
	Retinal haemorrhages
Toxoplasmosis	Uveitis, scleritis
Leishmaniasis	Anterior uveitis, keratitis, scleritis
Dirofilariasis	Anterior chamber worms, corneal oedema
Toxocariasis	Chorioretinitis
Diabetes mellitus	Rapidly developing cataract
	Diabetic retinopathy – retinal haemorrhages
Hypocalcaemia	Punctate and linear cataracts
Hyperadrenocorticism	Corneal ulceration, corneal lipidosis
Hypothyroidism	Corneal lipidosis, keratoconjunctivitis sicca
Lysozomal storage diseases	Faint corneal lipidosis
	Retinal deposits
Hypertension	Retinal haemorrhages
	Retinal detachment
Hyperlipidaemia	Corneal lipidosis, lipid keratopathy
	Lipaemia retinalis
Anaemia	Retinal haemorrhages
Thrombocytopaenia	Retinal haemorrhages
Hyperviscocity syndrome	Dilated tortous vessels
	Retinal haemorrhages
	Papilloedema
Vogt-koyanagi-harada syndrome	Anterior uveitis
	RPE and choroidal depigmentation
Lymphosarcoma	Anterior or posterior uveitis
	Retinal haemorrhages
Intracranial neoplasia	Papilloedema
	Blindness

Chapter 3

Adnexa and orbit

3.1 Lid laceration

Four key points should be taken into consideration when approaching the emergency case of a lid laceration.

1. Are there other ocular injuries? In many, if not the majority, of cases penetrating

globe injury also occurs and, given the haemorrhage and swelling accompanying lid trauma, such lacerations may be difficult to evaluate. However critical we consider lid injuries, a concurrent globe penetration is considerably more important from the viewpoint of potential long-term visual handicap. Missing such an injury is to be avoided at all costs.

2. When should surgery be undertaken? As we have said, there is often considerable lid swelling and haemorrhage associated with lid injury. As veterinarians we are often

---

Emergency management of lid lacerations

1. Perform full ophthalmic examination under sedation so as not to miss more severe globe trauma
2. If a very recent injury (less than 6 hours) repair immediately ensuring good lid margin apposition
3. If longer than 6 hours since injury bandage and give systemic NSAID, delaying repair until lid swelling has subsided
4. Always ensure that further self-trauma cannot occur by using Elizabethan collar, together with adequate analgesia

---

Prognostic indicators in lid lacerations

1. The profuse vascularization of the lid ensures that even substantial lacerations heal well
2. The key factor in ensuring adequate healing is adequate apposition of the lid margin to avoid long-term ocular surface irritation
3. Extensive damage and loss of tissue requiring reconstructive surgery

---

Eyelid injury in blunt trauma

1. Haemorrhage
2. Oedema
3. Important factor to look beyond the eyelid lesions to assess globe integrity, intra-ocular normality
4. The importance of shock-wave damage to tissue boundaries in the eye

---

Eyelid injury in sharp trauma

1. Laceration
2. Haemorrhage
3. Oedema
4. Critical: how much the tissue swelling compromises accurate re-apposition of lid edges?
5. If lids are well vascularized, tissues can be left protected, lubricated and clean for several days until swelling has reduced

tempted in such a situation to rush in with an immediate repair. This may often compromise our ability to perform an optimal repair. Assessing whether tissue is viable can be difficult in such circumstances, and ensuring that the lid margin is perfectly aligned may be impossible, given the degree of tissue swelling encountered. It may, in many cases, be preferable to protect the ocular surface with ointment, to provide a compress with a moistened bandage over the peri-orbital area and to treat with systemic non-steroidal anti-inflammatory agents for several days before attempting primary repair. This should be done only after thorough cleansing of the area. Systemic and local antibiotic therapy should be ensured. If the nasolacrimal system is damaged immediate primary repair may be deemed preferable or a nasolacrimal cannula can be sutured in place until repair is attempted. Once swelling has subsided and tissue viability can better be assessed a primary repair can be undertaken.

3. What tissue should be retained after a substantial injury and what removed? A strong temptation in lid repair is to preserve as much tissue as possible even where considerable damage has occurred. This may be counterproductive, as non-viable lid tissue will have to be removed in a secondary repair and subsequent problems of trichiasis or corneal exposure may occur. A preferable option is to remove substantially damaged tissue at primary repair and provide replacement tissue through skin rotation or bucket-handle flaps.

4. Finally, and perhaps most importantly, the repair of the lid margin in as near perfect apposition as possible is vital. An area of defective lid edge with associated trichiasis or the formation of a 'step' in the margin can give continual corneal problems and ocular surface irritation.

The correct placement of the first suture at the eyelid margin in a lid repair is thus critical in ensuring a successful result. A simple interrupted suture at the lid margin might be considered sufficient but in fact causes an unstable tissue union without adequate support. What is required is a cruciate (or

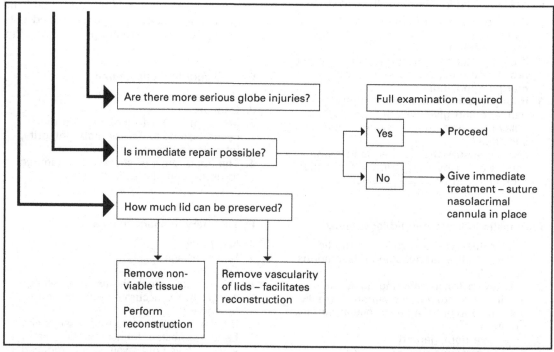

Box 3.1 Lid trauma

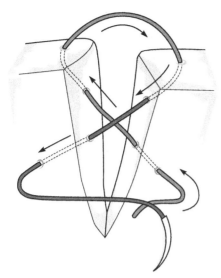

Figure 3.1 Suturing the lid margin

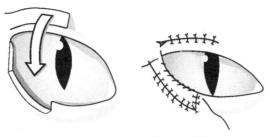

Figure 3.2 Reconstruction of lower lid from upper-lid with a skin flap

figure of 8) suture as shown in Figure 3.1. Starting at the external surface of the lid about 3 mm from the margin the suture is passed through the lid tissue and exits the lid at the margin. Re-entering the lid on the other side of the incision the suture again passes through the lid tissue to exit opposite the first suture entry-point. The suture thus firmly opposes the two parts of the lid both at the margin and at a point away from the lid edge. Single interrupted sutures of the lid skin oppose the edges of the lid incision, but beforehand sutures in the conjunctiva should be placed with their knots buried in the tissue of the conjunctiva.

A number of surgical options are available for long-term repair of substantial lid injury where tissue defects remain. These techniques are not really the subject for an emergency textbook but line diagrams illustrating the possible methods to remedy lid injuries with defects of upper and lower lids are given here (Figures 3.2–3.5).

3.2 Conjunctivitis

It might be objected that conjunctivitis cannot be considered an emergency: it is normally a chronic disease with an insidious onset, not causing overt pain or visual loss. Yet as a differential diagnosis for the red eye, and as a condition occasionally resulting in alarming chemosis and ocular discharge, it is right to

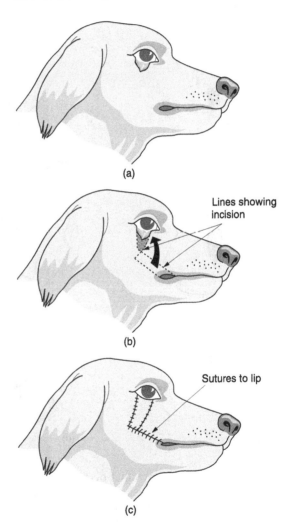

Figure 3.3 Pavletic lip-to-lid technique to reconstruct lower lid

include it here. Conjunctivitis can be caused by physical factors such as distichia or ectopic cilia (Helper and Magrane 1970); or entropion and trichiasis (Miller and Albert 1988); through

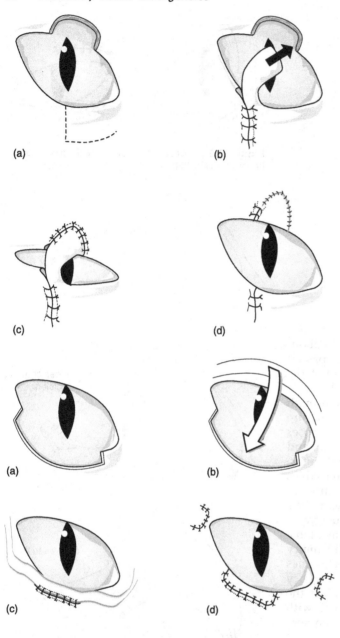

Figure 3.4 Reconstruction of upper lid defect from lower lid (Mustardé technique)

Figure 3.5 Bucket-handle techniques for lid defect

immunological pathways that occur in follicular conjunctivitis in dogs; or from infectious agents such as herpes virus, *Chlamydia* or *Mycoplasma* in cats (Nasisse et al. 1993). As such, conjunctivitis warrants a close ocular examination. In particular the bulbar aspect of the third eyelid should be examined. Often conjunctivitis persists even when the inciting cause of ocular irritation has been removed, because the lymphoid follicles which have formed on the bulbar surface of the nictitating membrane in response to chronic irritation are themselves a focus for ocular irritation. They should be removed by physical abrasion with

Differential diagnosis in conjunctival haemorrhage

- Ocular trauma
- Coagulopathy
- Systemic infections such as *Rickettsia rickettsiae*

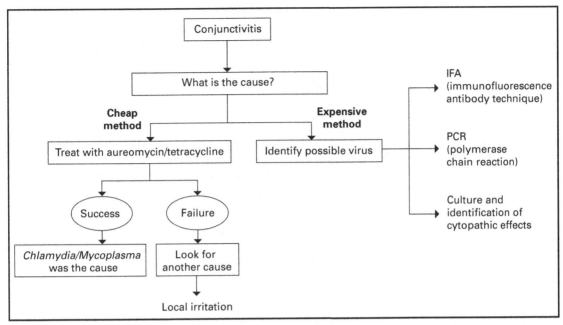

Box 3.2 Conjunctivitis

a cotton-tipped swab after topical anaesthesia, or in severe or refractory cases by the application of phenol, again with a cotton-tipped applicator (Dolowy 1987).

Conjunctivitis should never be treated initially with topical antibiotic with steroid medications. For one thing such polypharmacy reveals nothing about the possible causative agent even if the treatment has the desired effect. More importantly, in the cat, if the conjunctivitis is caused by ocular feline herpes virus infection, the steroid often has the effect of converting a mild harmless epithelial viral infection into a chronic sight-threatening corneal stromal infection with inflammation, neovascularization and refractory corneal oedema.

Feline keratoconjunctivitis may be caused by chlamydial or mycoplasmal as well as herpetic infection. Thus the use of topical tetracycline medication will have the effect of controlling the former two agents or, in the event of treatment failure, strongly suggesting viral infection to be the cause. In that case antiviral treatment may be considered to be the preferable course of action with diagnosis being achieved if such treatment is effective. A conjunctival scraping may be submitted for viral culture: for an immunofluorescent antibody (IFA) test to investigate the presence of *Chlamydia* and/or herpes virus, or for polymerase chain reaction (PCR) testing. In past years diagnosis of herpes viral infection was difficult and amelioration of signs on treatment was presumed to confirm diagnosis. Today with the availability of polymerase chain reaction-based diagnostic tests we can be more sure of a diagnosis of herpetic aetiology in feline keratoconjunctivitis. In the UK viral culture is most often used for diagnosis, but while the specificity here is high the sensitivity is poor with many false negative results. PCR testing is only available in the USA, while immunofluorescence is undertaken in Europe and is used by the two authors of this text residing on the eastern side of the Atlantic.

Treatment of FHV-1-related corneal disease can involve topical antiviral drops: idoxyridine (Herplex or Stroxil in USA) or trifluorothymidine (Viropticin USA or Moorfields Eye Hospital formulation in UK) drops four times daily. Topical interferon alpha (3000 IU/ml) has been used as has oral interferon (again 3000 IU/ml), 1 ml daily for seven days then alternating weeks. Other supportive but not curative treatment protocols include sytemic L-lysine (200–250 mg daily for the cat), and tear substitutes if tear production is reduced (Quinn 2000).

As the above-mentioned antiviral drugs are not widely available outside the USA, one of the authors (DLW) has successfully used a preparation of acyclovir (Zovirax ophthalmic), which is a licensed human ophthalmic ointment, for treatment of feline herpes virus keratitis even though the only paper on this subject showed poor antiviral effects *in vitro* (Nasisse et al. 1989). The results have so far been promising, but it is advisable to notify the owner that the drug is not licensed for veterinary use.

3.3 Dacryocystitis

An eye with severe frank purulent discharge may have a conjunctivitis but often the infection is related to a persistent infectious focus, either in the form of a foreign body or as dacryocystitis, where the infection centres in the nasolacrimal duct. In either of these cases examination under anaesthesia is often necessary: a full investigation of the depths of the conjunctival fornices should be undertaken to locate a foreign body such as a grass seed and the nasolacrimal duct should be flushed to assess the presence of dacryocystitis. In either case topical antibiosis should be provided but with dacryocystitis systemic medication is often needed and bacteriological culture and sensitivity are worthwhile to ensure that the correct drug is being used.

3.4 Conjunctival foreign body

The presentation of a non-penetrating conjunctival foreign body can be highly varied. Since foreign material can range from a grass awn to a piece of grit, signs occupy the whole spectrum from mild discomfort and purulent ocular discharge with the former to acute pain and chemosis with the latter. The key problem is finding such a foreign body in an eye where chemosis and adnexal swelling may easily hide the object. This is compounded by the tendency of many such foreign bodies to work their way into the fornix or to the very base of the third eyelid. This is especially true of grass awns.

In many cases the only way to investigate an eye where the possibility of a conjunctival foreign body is high is to examine the entirety of the conjunctival sac under general anaesthesia. Particular attention should be paid to the space behind the third eyelid and the full extent of the fornix around 360° of the globe. Copious irrigation will both clear any mucopurulent discharge which would otherwise obscure the view and also flush out small foreign bodies which might otherwise be missed.

3.5 Acute keratoconjunctivitis sicca

While keratoconjunctivitis sicca (KCS) might well be thought of as a chronic condition which would never be presented as an emergency, a small number of dogs with sudden-onset total failure of lacrimation present as acutely painful eyes with or without corneal ulceration. A considerable number of these cases, in the authors' experience, are the result of drug-induced KCS, mostly with salazopyrin use. Here the Schirmer tear test is zero and the whole ocular surface has a gritty appearance. It would appear, in our opinion, that these hyperacute failures of tear production are so severe because the conjunctiva has not had the opportunity to adjust its goblet-cell numbers and production of mucus. The classic mucopurulent ocular discharge so familiar in more chronic KCS is not seen in these cases, at least not in the first two to three weeks after emergency presentation. They do not seem responsive to management with topical cyclosporine although one might think that they should as lacrimal gland tissue has not been destroyed through a long-standing immune-mediated destruction (as occurs in the more chronic cases seen in the West Highland White terrier and Cocker spaniel).

Other cases of acute KCS include traumatic damage to the facial nerve or trigeminal damage resulting in reduced/absent corneal sensation and therefore reduced tear-production. In the former case there is often a dry nose, suggestive of denervation damage affecting the nasal glands which produce moisture at the external nares. In such neurological cases topical cyclosporine is less useful.

Even in cases of chronic dry eye the animal may be brought in as an emergency if a corneal ulcer supervenes. As will be discussed below one key feature in the investigation of a corneal ulcer is the determination of its cause: here a Schirmer tear test is just about obligatory to exclude KCS as a cause of the ulcer.

3.6 Exophthalmos

3.6.1 Globe protrusion or exophthalmos

This may be a gradually worsening disease or may be a sudden-onset emergency. It may signal a retrobulbar infection which can be relatively easily diagnosed and cured, or a retrobulbar neoplasm difficult to diagnose without recourse to expensive imaging techniques and often impossible to cure. Because of this dichotomy; the long-term damage to the eye from prolonged exposure; and, for the owner, the unpleasant appearance of the protruding globe it is important to manage these cases correctly from the start.

3.6.2 Orbital cellulitis and retrobulbar infection

The former may present as an acutely painful eye with a profuse mucopurulent ocular discharge or, if the infection has organized into an abscess, there may be the exophthalmos that occurs with a retrobulbar space-occupying mass, as discussed in section 3.6.3 below. Conjunctival hyperaemia is seen concurrent with the exophthalmos as may a serous or a mucopurulent discharge.

Retrobulbar infection often presents as exophthalmos associated with peri-apical dental disease – a tooth-root abscess may erupt as a open lesion on the skin or as a closed infected mass in the orbit producing globe protrusion.

The key feature in the diagnosis of such infective orbital disease is acute severe pain. Retropulsion of the globe is painful as is opening the mouth. This is important in assessment of the case as a fluctuant swelling may be detected behind the last molar tooth. Animals may be febrile and show signs of systemic malaise but this is not invariable. A haemogram is likely to reveal a neutrophilia.

Investigation of the area behind the last molar tooth should include an incision in the oral mucosa and gentle introduction of a closed haemostat into the orbit through the pterygoid muscle, followed by opening and withdrawal of the haemaostat, this obviously performed under general anaesthesia (Figure 3.6). While the literature would have one believe that 'purulent material usually drains from the affected area' (Speiss and Wallin-Håkanson 1999), in

---

Differential diagnosis in exophthalmos

Investigation should include
- Full ocular examination (including examination from above)
- Investigation of ocular movements (including forced retropulsion)
- Full cranial examination including opening mouth
- Ocular and orbital ultrasound
- Skull radiography and other imaging techniques (CT/MRI)

Causes
1. Retrobulbar mass
   - Abscess (painful on opening mouth)
   - Tumour (not generally painful on opening mouth)
2. Retrobulbar fluid
   - Oedema
   - Haemorrhage

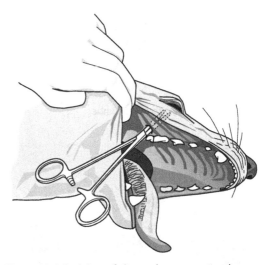

Figure 3.6 Incision of the oral mucosa, gentle introduction of a closed haemostat into the orbit through the pterygoid muscle followed by opening the haemaostat and withdrawal while animal is anaesthetized. Note that here the endotracheal tube and throat pack have been removed for sake of clarity, but should normally be used in such cases

our experience this is often not the case. We propose that the anatomy of the retrobulbar area often traps purulent material in lacunae but that drainage supported by aggressive systemic antibiotic treatment is almost always successful. Advancement of a bacteriological swab into the retrobulbar space can give useful culture data and the prevalence of anaerobes in a small series (DLW) supports the use of metronidazole together with a prolonged course of cephalosporin in these cases.

In rabbits and larger rodents such as the chinchilla the close apposition of the globe to the posterior dental molar roots leads to a range of problems, from the persistent epiphora often seen in chinchillas with dental disease to the frank severe exophthalmos seen in rabbits infected with *Pasteurella* or *Staphylococcus*. Dealing with this can be problematic since the extraction of infected teeth is difficult and yet without elimination of the focus of infection the condition cannot be remedied.

3.6.3 Other orbital space occupying lesions®

The gradually increasing exophthalmos occurring with a retrobulbar space-occupying lesion does not render it likely to be presented as an emergency, but three features here are important.

1. It will not be painful, as would the infected orbital cellulitis or retrobulbar abscess detailed above.
2. The exophthalmic globe should be differentiated from a hydrophthalmic, enlarged globe. The position of the nictitating membrane is important here: an exophthalmic globe will be characterized by a raised protuberant third eyelid while an enlarged globe, after severe glaucoma for instance, will not (Figure 3.7a–d).
3. The position of the retrobulbar space-occupying lesion, whether within the extra-ocular muscle cone (intraconal) or outside it (extraconal) substantially alters

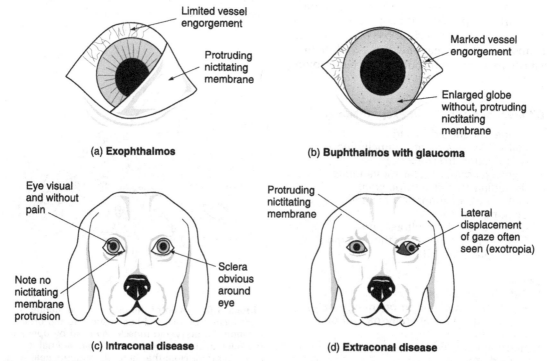

(a) **Exophthalmos**

Limited vessel engorgement

Protruding nictitating membrane

(b) **Buphthalmos with glaucoma**

Marked vessel engorgement

Enlarged globe without, protruding nictitating membrane

(c) **Intraconal disease**

Eye visual and without pain

Note no nictitating membrane protrusion

Sclera obvious around eye

(d) **Extraconal disease**

Protruding nictitating membrane

Lateral displacement of gaze often seen (exotropia)

Figure 3.7 Differentiating exophthalmos. (a) Exophthalmos; (b) enlarged globe; (c) Intraconial disease; (d) extraconial disease

the appearance of the eye. Intraconal disease leads to a staring appearance with sclera visible around the circumference of the cornea and, perhaps surprisingly, a lack of nictitating membrane protrusion (Figure 3.7). Intraconal disease may occur with an optic nerve tumour such as an intra-orbital menigioma but is more likely to occur acutely as an extra-ocular myositis (Ramsey et al. 1995, Ramsey and Fox 1997). In cases of eosinophilic extra-ocular myositis, leukocytosis and eosinophilia in a peripheral blood sample are seen and serum creatinine kinase levels are elevated.

Immunosuppressive doses of oral corticosteroids are usually ameliorative although azothioprine may also be valuable for two to three weeks at 1–2 mg/kg.

Other non-infectious space-occupying lesions do not of course have to be neoplastic. Masticatory myositis causes severe exophthalmos but also obvious signs of limited jaw movement, pyrexia, malaise and anorexia. Salivary retention cysts and mucocoeles can cause of slowly progressing extraconal exophthalmos which on draining yields a tenacious yellow fluid.

Chapter 4

Globe

4.1 Blunt trauma to the globe

Emergencies involving the entire globe are almost without exception traumatic. Penetrating injuries may involve the cornea or the sclera and are dealt with below. Blunt trauma

---

Emergency management of ocular contusion

1. Perform full ophthalmic examination, noting that damage may be as severe as with a penetratng injury
2. Perform fluorescein test to evaluate for surface ulceration
3. Measure intra-ocular pressure and treat accordingly
4. Give systemic corticosteroids and antibiotics
5. Give topical steroid if no corneal ulceration is present, otherwise give topical NSAID ketorolac (Acular, Allergan) or flurbiprofen (Ocufen, Allergan)
6. Give topical atropine twice daily
7. Hospitalize patient and evaluate eye every 3–4 hours

Prognostic indicators in ocular contusion

1. Intra-ocular haemorrhage is a poor prognostic sign
2. Intra-ocular inflammation is to be expected and can be ameliorated if treated aggressively
3. Glaucoma similarly may occur and is much less easily controllable than uveitis

---

to the globe might be considered less sight-threatening than penetrating injury but the shock waves that issue from severe blunt trauma can actually have more devastating effects than the localized injury resulting from penetrating trauma. A fracture of the bone surrounding the eye may similarly injure the globe and/or extra-ocular tissues.

In the same manner as an earthquake causes widespread disruption, the shock waves following blunt trauma have particularly catastrophic effects at boundaries between tissues with different physical characteristics (Figure 4.1). This is particularly seen at the iridocorneal angle where the connective tissues of the cornea and sclera meet the delicate soft tissue and vascular structures of the iris and ciliary body. The shearing forces following the shock waves resulting from a blunt traumatic episode cause irreversible tissue damage, separating the uveal structures from the connective tissue of the globe. Similarly the rebound forces occurring at the posterior face of the globe tear retina from choroid (or more correctly neurosensory retina from retinal pigment epithelium, given the potential space which exists between the two layers of the embryological optic cup). Such shearing forces may also tear vascular structures giving retinal or choroidal haemorrhages or vitreal haemorrhage arising from damage to the richly vascular ciliary body. Thus it can be seen that while penetrating trauma may itself cause significant local damage, blunt

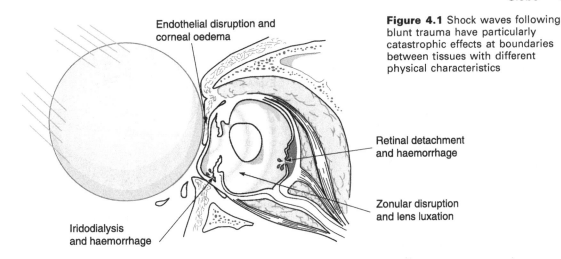

Endothelial disruption and corneal oedema

Iridodialysis and haemorrhage

Retinal detachment and haemorrhage

Zonular disruption and lens luxation

Figure 4.1 Shock waves following blunt trauma have particularly catastrophic effects at boundaries between tissues with different physical characteristics

trauma often gives rise to irreversible damage throughout the globe, even quite distant from the sight of blunt impact.

4.2. Globe prolapse

Perhaps the most acute ocular emergency, one for which treatment given within the first

---

> **Emergency management of the prolapsed eye**
>
> 1. Advise owner to attempt globe replacement in first minutes after injury with damp cotton wool pad
> 2. Advise owner to cover ocular surface with damp cotton wool pad while bringing to surgery
> 3. Administer shock dose of steroid i.v. (2 mg/kg)
> 4. Perform lateral canthotomy
> 5. Replace globe using only limited force – if more required enlarge canthotomy
> 6. Apply topical atropine and appropriate antibiotic (i.e. fusidic acid) ointment
> 7. Suture lids closed and leave for 10 days on systemic antibiotic and NSAID
>
> **Prognostic indicators in the prolapsed eye**
>
> 1. Extra-ocular muscle avulsion and strabismus gives a poor prognosis
> 2. Hyphaema with haemorrhage in the globe gives a poor prognosis as it suggests severe intra-ocular damage
> 3. The presence of a consensual light reflex is a good prognostic sign

few minutes after injury may be sight-preserving, is globe prolapse. This occurs predominantly in brachycephalic dogs in which globe exposure and a considerable degree of lagophthalmos is a natural phenomenon. The eyes are congenitally very exophthalmic and a frightening action such as a over-exuberant restraint of the neck region may cause prolapse of the globe.

Lateral trauma to the globe (the sort resulting from the animal's head being trapped in a closing door for instance) can result in globe prolapse in any breed. The entire globe is prolapsed beyond the lid margins. Here several pathological events occur (Figure 4.2). The optic nerve is obviously stretched, this potentially causing permanent visual loss. Vascular supply to the globe is compromised, with massive peribulbar tissue swelling and potentially disastrous effects on ocular health. Extra-ocular muscles may be damaged and avulsed from their globe origins, resulting in long-term strabismus.

In the time that it takes for an animal to be transported to the surgery the immediate trauma resulting from the prolapse will be compounded massively by the swelling occurring in the next few minutes. It is vital therefore to urge the owner to attempt to replace the globe behind the lids using a damp towel or piece of cotton wool placed on the globe surface, with a quite considerable degree of force exerted to replace the globe. As the inflammation is extensive, application of cold towels to the eye will reduce the swelling and act to prevent globe prolapse. In

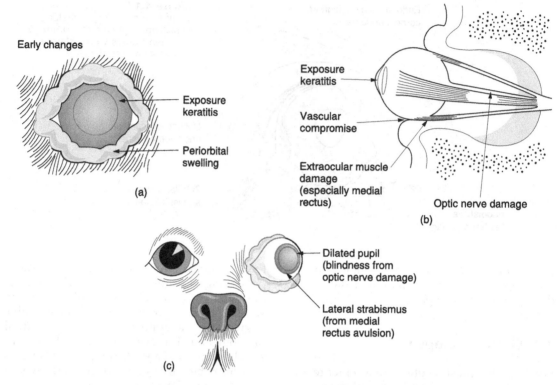

Figure 4.2 Pathological events in globe prolapse

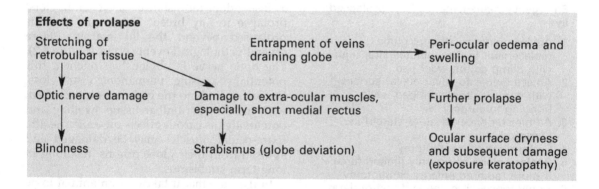

Effects of prolapse

Stretching of retrobulbar tissue	Entrapment of veins draining globe	Peri-ocular oedema and swelling
↓ ↘		↓
Optic nerve damage	Damage to extra-ocular muscles, especially short medial rectus	Further prolapse
↓	↓	↓
Blindness	Strabismus (globe deviation)	Ocular surface dryness and subsequent damage (exposure keratopathy)

Dealing with a globe prolapse (see Figure 4.2(d))

Immediate action	Retropulse globe into orbit if possible (before transport to hospital) Cover with wet swab or cotton wool (to prevent corneal dessication)
Definitive action	Give i.v. shock dose of dexamethasone Perform lateral canthotomy Replace globe Perform tarsorrhaphy and leave for 2–3 weeks
Long-term action	Give tear replacement if KCS occurs Resuture medial rectus muscle if lateral strabismus occurs

the first few minutes globe replacement is possible without surgery, but after this an extensive lateral canthotomy will be required to reposition the globe in the orbit because of the peribulbar conjunctival swelling occurring during this time. If the owner is not able to reposition the globe the animal should be transported to a veterinary centre with utmost urgency. The ocular surface must be protected and moistened to prevent surface drying and long-term damage before the globe can be surgically replaced in the orbit. A shock dose (2 mg/kg) of intravenous dexamethasone together with mannitol (1.0–1.5 g/kg) should be given slowly (an infusion pump delivering the total volume over 15–20 minutes is ideal) and will ameliorate the immediate after-effects of such a trauma.

After repositioning the globe a tarsorrhaphy should be performed. The eyelids should be re-opened only after several days. Only at that point can the eye be assessed to give an adequate prognosis regarding both return of vision and long-term cosmetic appearance; even if the eye will be non-visual a good emergency treatment will leave a cosmetically acceptable eye, and most owners will be satisfied and happy not to go through an enucleation. The prognosis will not in any case be particularly good unless the eye has been managed optimally in the critical period immediately after the prolapse.

Differential diagnosis in strabismus

- Full ophthalmic examination
- Investigation of passive ocular movement (including forced duction tests)
- Investigation of active ocular movement
- Full neurological examination

Strabismus may be caused by

- Retrobulbar mass
- Cranial nerve palsy (i.e. abducens or ocular motor involvement)
- Extra-ocular muscle trauma/fibrosis (post proptosis medial rectus damage)

4.3 Penetrating globe injury®

Suture patterns in the repair of globe lacerations are discussed in more detail under corneal lacerations: it is in the cornea that repairs require careful attention to ensure that transparency is maintained as much as possible. While iris prolapse occurs with disconcerting regularity through a corneal laceration, penetrating injury of the sclera clearly results more often in uveal trauma, given the anatomical proximity of the choroid to the sclera. Often in cats, having earlier had a laceration to the eye, the prolapse of a section of the iris would result in healing of the cornea, which may be observed at the annual booster. The eye is still visual but pupillary miosis and mydriasis are slightly impaired. The main problem with iridal prolapse through a corneal laceration – that is to say what tissue to resect as necrosed and non-viable – does not generally occur with a choroidal prolapse through a scleral wound. This is because the choroid usually bulges only to a limited extent through a scleral laceration. On the other hand the free pupillary edge of the iris can extend through a corneal laceration with vascular compromise, resulting in ischaemic necrosis of the iris on the external surface of the staphyloma. Thus while the difficult decision regarding the resection of such compromised and necrotic tissue has to be made for iris passing through a corneal laceration, the choroid exposed through a scleral laceration is generally healthier and easier to manage.

The problem posed by scleral laceration is one of infectious panophthalmitis. While one might be tempted, considering vascular compromise, to replace all exposed choroidal tissue back though a scleral laceration, the threat of intra-ocular infection and subsequent panophthalmitis is ever present. The danger is heightened by the fact that whatever caused the laceration must have passed into the eye, however briefly. As will be discussed below, lacerations at the limbus may be the result of blunt trauma, but scleral lacerations are normally direct injuries. This means that the lacerating agent may well have deposited some bacterial contamination in the posterior cavity. Unchecked, multiplication of such organisms can give rise to a fulminant panophthalmitis.

The question is then how to deal with such a laceration. Unless obviously necrotic it is advised that the choroid bulging through the laceration be replaced but only after a bacteriology swab of the exposed tissue has been taken and broad spectrum intravitreal and systemic antibiosis has been started. This is followed by medication specific to the organisms cultured from the bacteriological investigation. Swabbing for bacteriology may seem academically correct, but in the clinical setting intra-ocular deposition of antibiotics will be effective. Intra-ocular antibiotics may be used as detailed in Appendix C.

If compromised or necrotic choroid is to be removed, topical 1:1000 adrenaline should be applied to produce vasoconstriction and minimize bleeding from resected tissue. It is always better, as will be repeated with regard to iris presenting through a corneal laceration, to be more radical in removing healthy tissue at the edge of diseased uvea, than to be cautious and risk replacing tissue which will only act as a focus for necrosis and infection.

Chapter 5

Cornea

5.1 Corneal ulceration

Disruption of the integrity of the cornea may be divided into the following three categories (Schmidt 1977):

- Corneal erosion: disruption to the epithelial surface of the cornea without stromal damage
- Corneal ulceration: disruption of epithelium and a variable depth of corneal stroma
- Descemetocoele: disruption of corneal stroma to the level of Descemet's membrane with subsequent protrusion of elastic Descemet's membrane through stromal ulcer

Not all corneal ulcers present as emergencies. A logical approach to their diagnosis and treatment will aid in determining which are emergency cases. In any case the logical diagnostic protocol described below will allow evaluation of which therapeutic regimen is required for which particular ulcer type. Any reader who has had a corneal ulcer will be able to testify to the acute pain that may accompany such ocular surface erosion. For this reason, as well as the potential threat to globe integrity posed by a deep ulcer, corneal ulceration should always be viewed as a possible emergency situation.

Emergency management of deep corneal ulceration

1. Perform full ophthalmic examination
2. Define cause and depth of ulcer
3. If ulcer is small and mid depth consider performing radial keratotomy to promote stromal regeneration
4. If ulcer is small and deep perform conjunctival pedicle flap
5. If ulcer is larger and deep perform corneoscleral transposition
6. Provide protection through contact lens, nictitans flap or use porcine intenstinal submucosal graft

Prognostic indicators in corneal ulceration

1. Size and depth are critical factors in defining treatment success
2. Any evidence of stromal melting a poor prognostic sign
3. Any evidence of intra-ocular inflammation a poor prognostic sign

5.1.1 Is an ulcer present? – the use of ophthalmic stains

Corneal ulcers frequently present as a painful eye and as such the ocular surface of any painful eye should be closely examined to assess whether the epithelial surface is continuous or whether a discontinuity in the epithelial covering is present (Figure 5.1). In severe

Approach to the corneal ulcer

Initial full ophthalmic examination

↓

Perform Schirmer tear test

↓

Take bacteriology or virology swab if necessary

↓
    (i.e. if associated with purulent discharge
    or history of infected trauma
    or apparent FHV-1 infection)

Use fluorescein fully to delineate extent of ulcer

Questions to ask

1. What has caused the ulcer?
   - Exogenous trauma:
     physical injury
     chemical injury:
         acid
         alkali
         detergent
   - Internal factors
     basement membrane dystrophy
     KCS
     profound corneal oedema
2. How deep is the ulcer?
   - Superficial – involving epithelium only
   - Mid stromal
   - Deep stromal
   - Descemetocoele

3. Is the ulcer healing?
   - How long has it been present? (i.e. over seven days)
   - Is there a devitalized epithelial lip at the edge of a superficial ulcer?
   - Is there stromal vascularization?

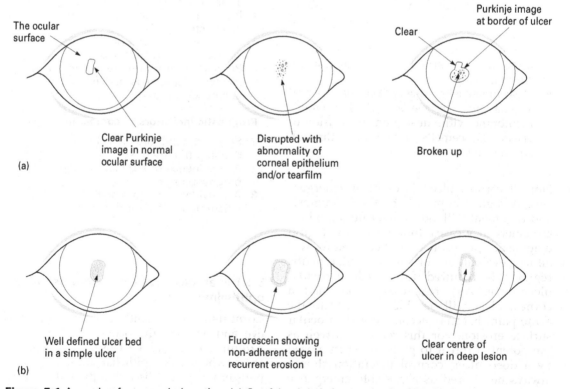

Figure 5.1 Assessing for corneal ulceration. (a) Careful ophthalmic examination; (b) the fluorescein test

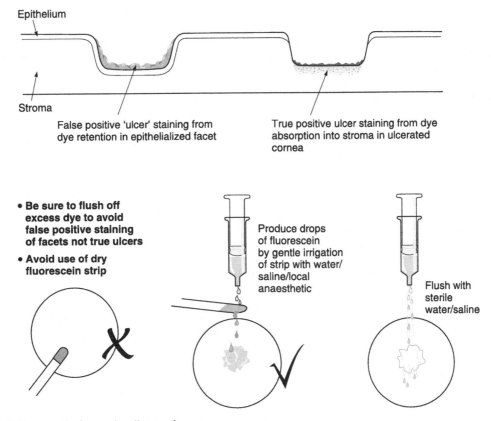

Epithelium

Stroma

False positive 'ulcer' staining from dye retention in epithelialized facet

True positive ulcer staining from dye absorption into stroma in ulcerated cornea

- **Be sure to flush off excess dye to avoid false positive staining of facets not true ulcers**

- **Avoid use of dry fluorescein strip**

Produce drops of fluorescein by gentle irrigation of strip with water/saline/local anaesthetic

Flush with sterile water/saline

Figure 5.2 Fluorescein for ocular diagnostic use

ulceration even a cursory examination will show a defect in the ocular surface but in superficial epithelial defects the lesion may easily be missed. Fluorescein is an invaluable diagnostic aid in such circumstances. Fluorescein for ocular diagnostic use may be applied using a fluorescein impregnated strip or fluorescein drops (see Appendix C). When using the strip some merely place the strip under the upper eyelid and use the tear film to dissolve and distribute the dye (Figure 5.2). A better method is to apply a drop or so of tear substitute or local anaesthetic to the strip before placing it gently on the ocular surface. This not only optimizes dye distribution but also will not cause any further ocular surface damage in an already compromised eye.

Whether this technique or a drop of fluorescein liquid is used, the diagnostic test should be attempted only after a Schirmer tear test has been performed. Tear evaluation should be the first diagnostic test in any

assessment of the ocular surface: other tests may well disturb the tear film and give erroneous Schirmer readings. Similarly corneal sampling for bacteriology, viral isolation or cytology should be carried out before the application of fluorescein. Topical anaesthetics should only be applied after bacteriology as some anaesthetics have been shown to be bacteriotoxic (Kleinfeld and Ellis 1966).

A key step in the fluorescein dye test is to flush away excess dye before examining the ocular surface. The irrigation of the eye with sterile water or saline using a syringe is ideal, although in an emergency a cotton wool pad soaked with water may be used to flush excess dye away. A minor but important precaution is a paper towel under the eye to keep dye away from clothing. For the same reason the animal's head should be well controlled.

Examination of the eye after staining is best performed with a blue light or by illumination with ultraviolet light from a Wood's fluorescent lamp. This may reveal subtle epithelial erosions which are much more difficult to examine with white light. A second advantage is that ulceration is so obvious with blue light that the owner can readily be shown the extent of the lesion, often not so easily appreciated with white light.

Fluorescein is an exceptionally polar molecule, and as such is excluded from the cornea by a healthy continuous epithelium with intact tight junctions between cells. The cornea is composed of hydrophobic epithelium and stroma Fluorescein, being hydrophilic, does not penetrate the epithelium but will penetrate the stroma when a superficial ulcer is present. The extent of the coloration must be assessed shortly after application, as the dye can diffuse both vertically and horizontally, giving a false impression of the area involved (Gelatt 1978). In the Boxer indolent ulcers dye diffuses quickly under the epithelial flap, but this is normally obvious given the clear edge of the ulcer. Any defect in the epithelium, allowing water to pass from the tear film to the stroma, will be revealed by fluorescein which moves with the water into the stroma, instead of being flushed away by ocular surface irrigation. This is why good flushing of the eye is important: a slight surface irregularity in which epithelium is still intact and not ulcerated may otherwise appear to pick up stain just because the dye is pooling in these surface epithelial irregularities. Such an irregularity is called a pit or a facet, where an ulcer has previously caused a defect in the stromal thickness, later being covered by intact epithelium.

Rose bengal was previously thought to stain devitalized corneal tissue. It is now used for staining the ocular surface when the mucin layer of the precorneal tear film is deficient (Feenstra and Tseng 1992): this occurs in situations where the epithelial surface is compromised, but not perhaps completely obliterated. If the epithelial barrier is not destroyed fluorescein will not stain. Thus rose bengal is useful to stain partial thickness epithelial defects. Such ulcers occur in ulcerative feline herpes keratitis before complete thickness epithelial ulcers are seen stained with fluorescein. The theoretical disadvantage of using rose bengal is that it is reported as being painful when used in people. In our experience, cats in which the stain has been used do not generally show any signs of discomfort such as blepharospasm. Other drugs such as tropicamide can be a quite severe irritant for a few seconds in humans but do not seem to illicit similar signs in companion animals. It is not therefore considered inappropriate to use such a drug routinely in dogs and cats.

5.1.2 Three key questions regarding any corneal ulcer (see Figure 5.3)

- How deep is the ulcer?
- Is the ulcer healing adequately?
- Why is there are ulcer there is the first place?

The first two questions are in many ways linked as will be seen below, but here each will be taken separately.

5.1.2.1 Ulcer depth Regarding the depth of the lesion, ulcers can be classified as being superficial, partial thickness or descemetocoeles. In this classification superficial ulcers really involve only epithelial erosion without stromal destruction. Partial thickness ulcers have stromal extension of epithelial defects and this can run from margin stromal involvement to deep ulceration. Descemetocoeles form when all stromal tissue has been destroyed, leaving only Descemet's membrane. This, being elastic in nature because of its collagen type IV content, bulges through the stromal defect under intra-ocular pressure.

How are these different depths of ulcer to be differentiated? Close examination, ideally with a slit lamp but more usually in an emergency situation with a magnifying loupe or direct ophthalmoscope at +20 D as described above, shows the depth of ulcer clearly merely by the appearance of the ulcer edge; but some further clues aid evaluation. The first is the degree of stromal oedema associated with the ulcer. A superficial epithelial erosion will have little or no stromal oedema, simply because the stroma has had little opportunity to imbibe water and has not undergone tissue damage. A partial thickness ulcer will have a varying

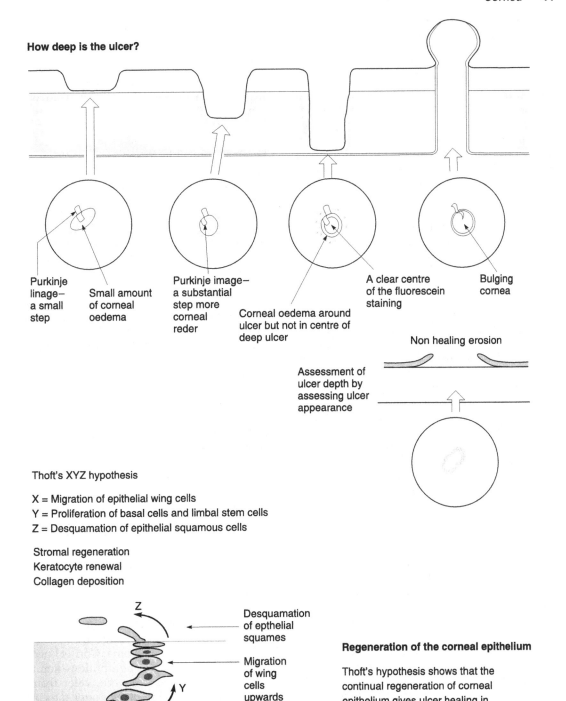

How deep is the ulcer?

Purkinje linage—
a small step

Small amount of corneal oedema

Purkinje image—
a substantial step more corneal reder

Corneal oedema around ulcer but not in centre of deep ulcer

A clear centre of the fluorescein staining

Bulging cornea

Assessment of ulcer depth by assessing ulcer appearance

Non healing erosion

Thoft's XYZ hypothesis

X = Migration of epithelial wing cells
Y = Proliferation of basal cells and limbal stem cells
Z = Desquamation of epithelial squamous cells

Stromal regeneration
Keratocyte renewal
Collagen deposition

Z

Desquamation of epthelial squames

Migration of wing cells upwards

Y

Basal cell multiplication to create wing cells

X

Basal cells migrating from limbal stem cell population

Regeneration of the corneal epithelium

Thoft's hypothesis shows that the continual regeneration of corneal epithelium gives ulcer healing in around 7 days when X + Y = Z. Any bigger and a cause for delayed healing should be sought.

Figure 5.3 Key questions to ask of an ulcer

degree of stromal oedema around it depending on how much excess water has been taken up by stromal tissue. This involves the centre of the ulcer and also a halo of cornea around the lesion. Most important is the deep ulcer, which may have considerable peri-ulcerative oedema but in which the centre of the ulcer is clear of oedema, often manifesting quite a bright appearance because of tapetal reflectivity through the remaining corneal tissue. In fact the clarity of tapetal reflection, in contrast to the surrounding stromal oedema, shows that the ulcer has all but completely perforated the corneal stroma. These ulcers are real emergencies, as a little more stromal destruction will lead to a descemetocoele. The descemetocoele is generally easy to recognize since the clear Descemet's membrane protrudes through the surrounding stroma to some extent, producing a dome-like structure in the midst of considerable oedematous stromal opacity.

5.1.2.2 *Ulcer healing* The degree of healing

response of the cornea around the ulcer should be determined to give a full evaluation of the corneal ulcer. Each of the above classes of ulcer depth can be assessed for signs of healing.

The superficial corneal ulcer or erosion which is going to heal will have done so, or at the very least shown a significant reduction in ulcer size, within three to five days, given adequate corneal protection. The superficial ulcer which is not going to heal this rapidly will be characterized by a lip of non-healing devitalized non-adherent epithelial tissue. The deeper stromal ulcer which is in the process of healing will show a gradual epithelialization of the ulcer crater within the first few days, eventually leaving a fully epithelialized corneal facet. Such a healing ulcer will also be characterized by vascular ingrowth from the limbus. The problem is not, perhaps, so much one of not healing, but of healing that is not progressing rapidly enough or filling in the stromal deficit completely enough. Given the propensity of such ulcers to deepen further it is important to treat them as if they were liable to perforate at any moment. It is with these ulcers that the third question must be answered quickly: what is the reason for the ulcer? The answer is likely to show also what is causing

progression in ulcer depth and what can be changed to remedy the situation.

5.1.2.3 *The aetiology of the ulcer* The

primary reason for ulcer formation may arise from within the cornea itself or from within the rest of the ocular apparatus, or there may be an external infectious or external physical cause. The prime case of a corneal defect itself being responsible for ulcer formation is the epithelial basement membrane dystrophy discussed below. Here in fact the dystrophy may not be responsible for the initial ulcer formation but is the underlying defect which prevents rapid healing of a minor erosion which might, in a normal cornea, not even cause enough of a problem to necessitate the animal being presented to a veterinarian.

Abnormalities in the rest of the eye fall into several groups. Lid defects may give rise to corneal abrasions in several conditions. Entropion and post-traumatic lid defects in any breed, or congenital abnormalities such as the lid colobomas in cats, can all lead to trichiasis where normal hair abrades the corneal surface. The same can be seen when a skin fold in a brachycephalic breed causes normal hair to contact the cornea. Medial canthal lashes can cause a similar problem and, being short and stubby, these can result in considerable corneal pathological changes, either as aberrant pigmentation and keratitis, or a corneal ulcer. Similarly distichiasis, with aberrant cilia from the meibomian gland openings, or an ectopic cilium from a conjunctival hair follicle, can cause corneal abrasion resulting in a corneal ulcer. A neurological deficit such as a facial paralysis can cause an exposure keratopathy which may well include corneal ulceration.

Other intrinsic defects that can lead to corneal ulceration include conditions causing corneal oedema. These range from endothelial dystrophies to glaucoma. Corneal oedema leads to ulceration through bullous keratopathy. When oedema is severe water from the stroma can extrude in blebs under the corneal epithelium, with formation of epithelial bullae. These are prone to burst, either spontaneously or with the slightest of external forces, giving rise to a corneal ulcer. The difficulty is that the underlying corneal oedema renders healing problematic: spontaneous healing is unlikely to occur and techniques used to promote epithelial healing with a normal stroma often fail to work in the face of stromal oedema. More promising methods are discussed in section 5.2.2.

An important intrinsic cause of ulceration is keratoconjunctivitis sicca (KCS). A deficiency in the all-important lubricating tear covering of the ocular surface is a common factor in the genesis of corneal ulceration. KCS may be the root of chronic ulcerative problems but can also result in acute and very painful surface ulceration. KCS as an underlying problem shows the importance of fully investigating the eye before attempting to treat the ulceration. Any therapeutic regimen attempted in the presence of a dry eye will fail. Amelioration of tear deficiency, either with tear replacement or better with topical cyclosporine, may allow ulcer healing with little in the way of intensive ocular surface management.

It might seem surprising that discussion of infection as a predisposing cause of corneal ulceration has not been considered earlier in this list of causes of corneal ulceration. Corneal Gram-negative or fungal infection may be an important complicating factor in corneal ulceration but bacterial or fungal agents are not particularly common as predisposing factors in corneal ulceration. Viral disease is a prime cause but such virally mediated ulcerations are recognized with certainty only in the cat. Here feline herpes virus is the primary cause of dendritic, and possibly also geographic, ulceration. Equine herpes virus is thought to have a similar role in the horse but definitive evidence for this is lacking. A number of cases of punctate ulceration occur in the dog, and given the prevalence of similar ulceration in man with an adenoviral aetiology, a viral cause may occur here although none has been determined to date.

Finally, trauma is at the root of many corneal ulcers, with or without other complicating factors as discussed above. Traumatic incidents, from superficial abrasions to deep wounds, would be relatively easy to treat but for the addition of complicating factors from inherited corneal defects to external

---

Treating the corneal ulcer

The assumption is made that any predisposing cause has been addressed

- The healing superficial ulcer: antibiotic cover using chloramphenicol drops or other antibiotics

- The non-healing superficial ulcer:
    protection:
        therapeutic contact lens
        third eyelid flap
        tarsorraphy
    debridement:
        removal of devitalized epithelium with dry swab or scalpel blade
        alteration of ulcer bed: punctate or grid keratomy
        or by partial thickness keratectomy
    analgesia:
        use of systemic NSAID such as oral carprofen

- The stromal ulcer less than 1/2 corneal depth
    protection:
        therapeutic contact lens
        third eyelid flap ⎤ not recommended as deepening of ulcer
        tarsorraphy   ⎦ will be more difficult to recognize

- The deeper stromal ulcer or descemetocoele
        conjunctival pedicle flap
        corneoscleral transposition

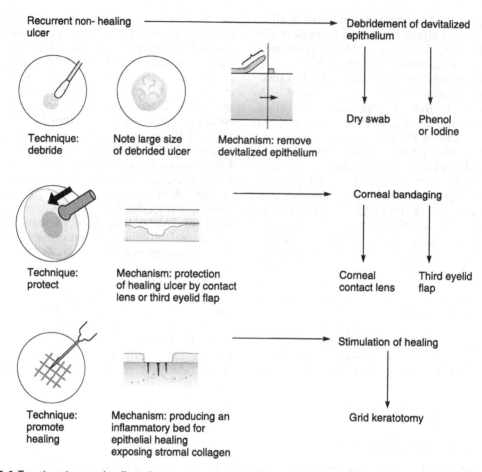

Box 5.1 Treating the non-healing ulcer

infections. In section 5.2 we consider the management of the different forms of ulcer described above. Only when the ulcer has been fully assessed for depth, healing and aetiology can one be happy to proceed with the correct course of ulcer management.

5.2 Dealing with different ulcers

5.2.1 The simple healing superficial ulcer

A superficial erosion with solely epithelial or epithelial and only superficial stromal involvement can be effectively managed with topical antibiosis and re-examined in five days, as long as no intrinsic or infectious cause is determined. In such a case topical antibiosis with fucidic acid in the dog or topical chlortetracycline in the cat would be appropriate. Within this time a non-complicated ulcer will have healed. Any persistence of ulceration would call for re-appraisal of the ulcer and possible recategorization of the lesion as a persistent ulcer, as discussed above.

5.2.2 The recurrent or persistent non-healing superficial ulcer

Healing response is particularly important in gauging the superficial ulcer. While some of these ulcers will occur as a result of trauma to a healthy cornea many of them will be refractory, recurrent ulcers in which healing is not occurring as it should. This generally occurs for one of three reasons. The first and best recognized is true epithelial basement membrane dystrophy. The second is severe corneal oedema where cystic blebs arise from stromal excretion of water giving a bullous keratopathy. The third is less than optimal healing in an older animal. These three conditions will be discussed further below.

The most common condition resulting in a non-healing ulcer is that occurring in dogs with epithelial basement membrane dystrophic change: here there is a diminution in the number of hemidesmosomes, the anchoring points by which the basal epithelial cell complex attaches to the underlying stroma. These ulcers are seen in Boxer dogs and Pembroke corgis particularly although recently a number of West Highland White terriers have been seen by one of us with similar disease.

The classic recurrent ulcer has a lip of devitalized epithelium around the edge of the ulcer. This prevents the healthy corneal epithelium migrating to the ulcer edge and commencing the healing response. Thus the first step in any therapeutic protocol for such ulcers must be to remove this dying non-adherent epithelium, as described further below.

Disturbance of the ocular surface with a dry swab or with a piece of cotton wool wrapped around a fine haemostat will peel off this poorly adherent epithelium, confirming the diagnosis of epithelial basement

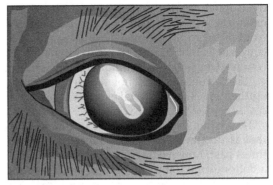

Box 5.2 Devitalized epithelium becomes white after phenol cautery

membrane dystrophy. The technique of epithelial debridement is for that reason important diagnostically as well as therapeutically.

Determining healing is equally, if not more, important for deeper ulcers involving the stroma. Here a key feature indicating a vigorous healing response is the invasion of blood vessels from the limbus to the ulcer edge. A firm grasp of the pathophysiology of corneal ulcer healing requires considerable understanding of the mechanisms at work in both epithelial and stromal healing, as presented below.

Removal of all devitalized, poorly adherent epithelium is vital to allow full healing of

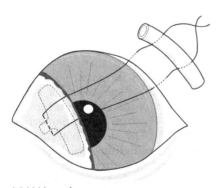

(a) Lid-based

(b) Conjunctiva-based

Note in each case:

- anchoring around the third eyelid cartilage
- different entry of suture into third eyelid
- two sutures may be needed in many cases

Figure 5.4 Third eyelid flap anchoring to (a) upper eyelid; (b) episclera

dystrophic epithelial erosions. Often quite extensive amounts can readily be stripped from a dystrophic cornea. One should not be concerned that normal epithelium will be removed by such a technique. Even quite a vigorous rubbing will not disturb a healthy epithelium while it takes little effort to dislodge devitalized tissue.

Today this dry debridement is generally all that is documented in the standard texts. In times past, however, agents such as phenol on a cotton tipped applicator were used to good effect and might be considered appropriate, if not actually preferable, to dry debridement. As with the latter technique phenol does not damage healthy epithelium and so is usefully selective of dystrophic epithelial tissue.

In some cases debridement and corneal bandaging are all that is necessary to promote full healing. In cases where this fails a number of treatment regimens have been reported on. It is generally the case that where several treatment options exist one can assume that none is universally successful. This is the case with persistent recurrent erosions: the best treatment for these ulcers is difficult to determine. The very terms recurrent, persistent and recidivistic strongly suggest that achieving full permanent healing is not easy. Given the failure of any one technique to give acceptable results in every case it will be worthwhile to consider the different options for treatment.

The basic science behind the different treatment regimens should be understood to facilitate treatment planning. We have already discussed measures to remove devitalized epithelial tissue from the path of new epithelial cell migration. The second important feature in a therapeutic plan should be to minimize trauma to the epithelial surface during healing. In her comparative survey of treatment methods, Susan McLaughlin determined that of all the options the most successful, either alone or in combination with other methods, was the third eyelid flap. Today we might prefer to provide a corneal bandage using a therapeutic contact lens. This has the advantage that the eye can both see and be seen but the disadvantage that, while the nictitating membrane flap will be secure until released, a contact lens may not stay in place for ten or so days until full corneal healing has taken place.

If a third eyelid flap is to be placed one of two techniques can be used, each favoured by different groups of ophthalmologists (Figure 5.4). Some say that the third eyelid should be secured not to the lid but to the bulbar conjunctiva. This ensures that when the eye moves so does the flap. When secured to the lid there is always the possibility of some friction between the flap and the cornea as the globe moves. This is probably very slight but in destabilized ocular surface problems it is wise to take every step possible to minimize even mild surface trauma. Nevertheless other ophthalmologists prefer anchoring the third eyelid to the upper eyelid, since if long ends are left to the sutures the flap can be released and then repositioned without the need to anaesthetize the animal again.

Removing diseased tissue and protecting the corneal surface are the bare essentials of treatment for such persistent erosions. As has been suggested a considerable proportion of these ulcers will heal with this treatment alone. The rationale for subsequent treatments is either to disrupt the epitheliostromal boundary with its basement membrane or to provoke a considerable superficial stromal scarring effect. The first retains good vision at the end of the treatment period while the latter tends to give scar formation reducing visual acuity considerably. Such treatments should be used either when the eye is already blind or when nothing else will work. The former rationale is the basis for the techniques of grid or punctate keratotomy. The latter is the reason behind the thermal keratoplasty described below.

Grid keratotomy uses a 21–23 gauge needle to produce, as its name suggests, a grid of lines over the ulcerated area while punctate keratotomy merely produces pinpoint punctures in the most superficial stroma (Figure 5.5). The aim of both these techniques is that the epithelium which grows down into the gridline or puncture points should serve to anchor the whole epithelial sheet in place. For this reason the gridlines or punctures do not need to be as close together as when the aim is to disturb the whole basement membrane surface. The technique can be undertaken in the conscious dog with topical anaesthesia and perhaps mild sedation in a nervous or boisterous individual. In a matter

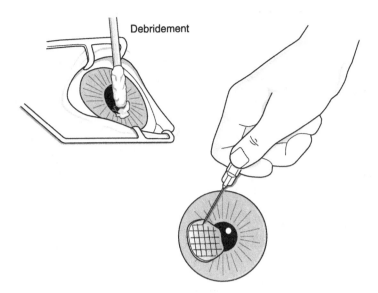

Debridement

Figure 5.5 Debridement and grid keratomy for an indolent ulcer

of a few days epithelial healing occurs after such a keratotomy, although in many cases accompanied by considerable vascularization. This can be removed once full ulcer healing has occurred by the use of topical steroids. Many ophthalmologists rightly feel that using steroids in an eye predisposed to ulceration is unwise. Steroids markedly impair epithelial healing and, were a subsequent ulcer to occur, the use of these agents would be most definitely contra-indicated. The advent of readily available topical non-steroidal anti-inflammatory drugs such as flurbiprofen or diclofenac has on the whole rendered unnecessary the use of steroids to reduce post-healing vascularization of the ulcer bed.

5.2.3 Ulceration secondary to bullous keratopathy®

In recurrent ulceration secondary to bullous keratopathy in corneal oedema, techniques such as the keratotomies often fail to work. Here a technique to produce epitheliostromal scarring can be used, where the eye has little vision in any case. In thermal keratoplasty a thermocautery tip produces spot-welds in the cornea with about the same distribution as the stromal punctures in punctate keratotomy, that is leaving a distance of about 1 mm between applications (Wilkie and Whittaker 1997) (Figure 5.5). Some ophthalmologists perform this without stripping the overlying

epithelium while others thoroughly debride the ocular surface first.

5.2.4 Partial thickness stromal ulceration

Ulcers with stromal involvement may be managed conservatively if they are less than one third of the corneal thickness in depth. The decision whether to leave the ulcer to heal or to perform a grid keratotomy or a superficial lamellar keratectomy is often difficult. If the ulcer is extensive and re-epithelialization of the cornea has not occurred, a debridement including grid keratotomy or lamellar keratectomy can be used. Grid keratotomy can be performed under local anaesthesia. It is important to rest the hand with the needle on the face inferior to the eye, so if the animal suddenly moves (which is most often drawing the head back) a penetration of the globe will not happen. The use of bandage contact lenses may be preferred over performing a third eyelid flap, for it is in these partial thickness ulcers that regular monitoring is essential to ensure that the ulcer is healing rather than becoming deeper. If epithelialization of a partial thickness ulcer is progressing, this shows that healing is occurring and in most cases, where there is still some considerable thickness of corneal stroma intact, careful observation can be appropriate.

- Is the cornea perforated?
    The Seidel test showing a perforation:
        dry the cornea
        apply drop of fluorescein (uniform yellow colour)
        watch for 'snaking' stream of aqueous from the laceration

- Is there prolapse of iridal tissue?
    Evaluate the health of protruding iris for 24 hours the surface covering of exuded serum protects iris, thus a substantial number of staphylomas can be replaced. 'If it bleeds it is not too compromised' is a useful maxim

- Aim to replace as much non-infected recently traumatized tissue as possible

- Use visco-elastic gel to break down iridocorneal adhesions

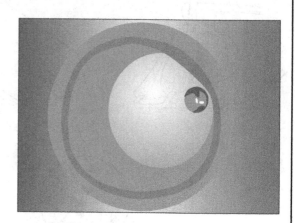

Box 5.3 Treating the perforated cornea

A progressing ulcer one over a third of the corneal thickness in depth or a descemeto-coele where the ulcer has breached the entire thickness of the stroma should all be considered as urgent emergencies and treated with conjunctival pedicle flaps or possibly with Gaiddon's technique of radial keratotomy (Gaiddon 1996), as discussed further in this section.

In the case of a partial thickness ulcer which is not showing any signs of healing, there are perhaps three therapeutic options available. The first is to perform a conjunctival pedicle flap as described in section 5.2.5. This has the great advantage that it ensures a result which is watertight and also allows serum from the cut surface of the pedicle flap to seep continually into the underlying ulcerated stroma providing both growth factors and collagenase inhibitory alpha 2 macroglobulins. It does, however, give a significant obstruction to vision, often in the primary line of sight. The conjunctival flap may not always be the perfect choice of treatment for a midstromal ulcer but it is a safe method, where the veterinary clinician is at little risk of perforating the globe. Thus the authors recommend the conjunctival flap as a safe surgical treatment which may cause some scarring of the cornea postoperatively.

A second option, regularly used in human ophthalmology but employed less frequently in the veterinary field, is the use of cyano-acrylate glue in the stromal wound (Figure 5.6).

Use of butyl cyanoacrylate glue requires

- an anaesthetized patient with an immobilized eye
- a completely dry corneal surface. The best way of ensuring this is to use a photographer's drying gas aerosol over the surface of the cornea
- a well controlled application of a small amount of glue painted onto the ulcer bed with a fine (25 G) needle (Figure 5.7).

5.2.5 Near-penetrating ulcers, descemetocoeles and penetrating ulcers®

As noted above an ulcer which is at the point of penetrating or has developed a descemeto-coele should be taken to surgery urgently. Even if perforation does occur during surgery, it is clearly much to be preferred that such an entry into the anterior chamber should occur in the controlled sterile environment of the operating theatre rather than in a home or field setting.

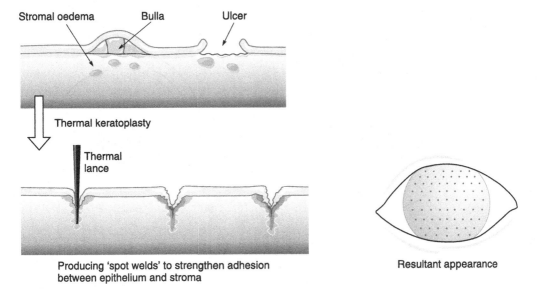

Figure 5.6 Bullous keratopathy – pathogenesis and treatment

The optimal technique for performing a conjunctival pedicle flap is shown in Figure 5.8. A pinch of conjunctiva is taken around 5 mm from the limbus and a pair of tenotomy scissors used to incise the conjunctiva and then bluntly dissect under the conjunctival epithelium. It is easy to achieve a single plane of dissection if the whole flap is prepared by blunt dissection through one small keyhole incision. Making a larger

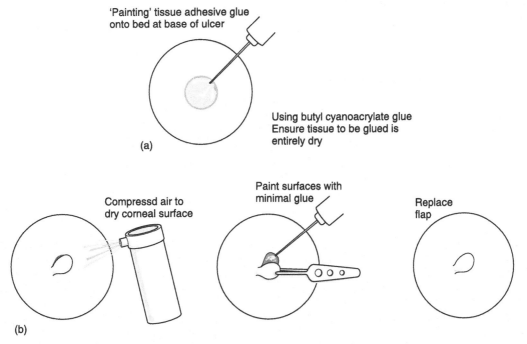

Figure 5.7 Painting glue onto the ulcer bed

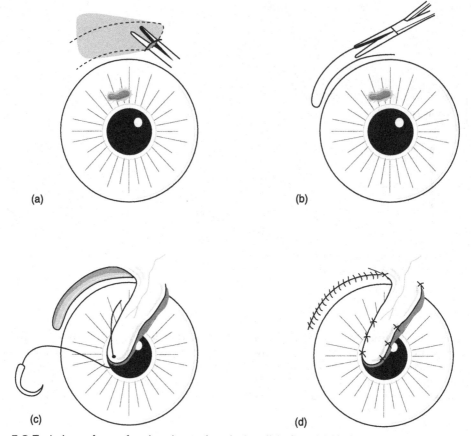

Figure 5.8 Techniques for performing the conjunctival pedicle flap. (a) Undermine conjunctiva from one entry point; (b) cut flap with base opposite ulcer; (c) position flap; (d) suture flap and close

Performing the conjunctival pedicle flap

Reasons: Deep corneal ulcer   Melting ulcer   Descemetocoele

Mechanism: Immediate physical repair of defect
                      Source of serum with immunoglobulins and macroglobulins

For the technique, see Figure 5.8.

incision early in the procedure results in a number of planes of dissection and generally gives a thicker and less ideal flap. The flap should be thin enough to be moved easily around and stretched over the ulcer bed. Always make the flap square and larger than the ulcer so it can be trimmed to fit the defect. It should be sutured in place with a fine absorbable suture such as 6/0 or better still 8/0 vicryl. The neck of the pedicle should be left unsutured so that when the ulcer has healed the pedicle can be divided, leaving a small island of conjunctiva which, deprived of blood supply, will eventually be incorporated into a small corneal scar, allowing vision even when in the visual axis.

An alternative technique is that of Jacques Gaiddon using the radial keratotomy technique perfected for the treatment of human myopia (Gaiddon 1996). Gaiddon reasoned that since the basis of radial keratotomy for myopia was the induction of stromal remodelling, and this was just what was needed in deep stromal ulceration, deep radial keratotomy would be appropriate in deep ulceration in the dog. This certainly works, with substantial reduction in depth of the ulcer and eventual complete healing, but has yet to be taken up by veterinary ophthalmologists in any great number.

5.2.6 The melting ulcer®

5.2.6.1 The melting ulcer: diagnosis The signs of a melting, or collagenolytic, corneal ulcer are obvious at clinical presentation. Where a normal stromal ulcer may have considerable corneal oedema or vascular and cellular infiltrate, its edge is relatively well defined and the surrounding stroma appears predominantly healthy. The melting ulcer has, as its name suggests, an appearance of progressing from the tectonically structured solid stroma to an almost fluid consistency. While oedema gives a ground-glass appearance to the cornea such stromal lysis often produces a much more dense white opacification of the stroma. The collagen fibrils which are the support structures in the stroma are broken down by a variety of enzymes resulting in degraded stroma which in many cases is so fluid as gradually to run from the ocular surface down the eyelid. These collagenolytic enzymes may be derived from bacteria such as *Pseudomonas* or from polymorphonucleocytes infiltrating infected cornea. It is the presence of bacteria producing the enzymes and the action of the enzymes which must be considered in formulating the diagnostic and therapeutic plan.

In the horse a recent report (Brooks et al. 2000) described melting ulcers being caused by Streptococci, demonstrating that it is important not to assume that a melting ulcer is caused by *Pseudomonas* and thus only applying aminoglycosides. These antibiotics may have little if any action on staphylococci and streptococci, thus aggravating the problem.

A bacteriology swab should be taken as discussed above and cultured with urgency. A smear of such a swab on a couple of microscope slides allows one to be stained with Gram's method and the other with lactophenol cotton blue and immediate evaluation of whether a Gram-positive or, more likely, a Gram-negative or fungal agent is responsible. A corneal scraping under local anaesthetic and/or sedation should also be undertaken and the scraping applied directly to a blood agar plate for immediate inoculation. Even before the full result of these bacteriological investigations is known treatment must be instituted with haste as discussed in section 5.2.6.2.

The anamnesis of the case as well as the characteristics of previous disease in the geographical area are important in a full evaluation of the disease. In some areas particular organisms are more common that others and this, together with information regarding the involvement of, say, an injury with possibility of a plant material corneal foreign body, is important in the full investigation of such an ulcer.

5.2.6.2 The melting ulcer: treatment Frequent – initially hourly – application of a broad spectrum antibiotic with action against the bacteria most likely to be causing this collagenolysis – predominantly *Pseudomonas* and *Proteus* – is very important. Previously, as discussed above, this meant the use of topical gentamicin but drug resistance in many cases has led to changes. Fortified preparations, with powder for intravenous gentamicin use, dissolved in artificial tears or in a topical base have been recommended. Recently in the UK a formulation of gentamicin with EDTA and trometamol has been licensed. The EDTA is not likely to be at a sufficient dose for efficacy in collagenase inhibition (see below in this section) but it does increase the efficacy of the gentamicin by facilitating drug uptake by bacteria. Trometamol also increases drug absorption by bacteria and thus similarly raises drug efficacy. More recently available drugs include the quinolones, but although these are effective against Gram-negative organisms their use in veterinary ophthalmology has yet to be assessed fully (Figure 5.9).

A diagnostic and therapeutic approach

History   – often history of trauma
             – possible involvement of plant or other organic material
             – rapid deterioration in corneal condition
Appearance – white/cream ill-defined corneal opacity
             – irregular corneal surface
             – frank corneal liquefaction
             – ocular pain

Treatment

(i)   Sedation (and/or peri-ocular nerve blocks in the horse)
(ii)   Take swabs and scrapings from affected cornea, including lesion edge cytology – Gram and Diff
       Quick stains for immediate presumptive identification of infectious organisms' culture and sensitivity
       – both bacterial and fungal
(iii) Insert subpalpebral or nasolacrimal medication device
(iv)   Apply antibiotic and anticollagenolytic medication hourly to start
       Antibiotics   fluoroquinolones (Exocin (Allergan))
                            fortified preservative-free antibiotic solution

Drug	Commercially available strength	Suggested fortified strength	Shelf-life
Amikacin		10 mg/ml	30 days
Carbenicillin		4–8 mg/ml	3 days
Gentamicin		3 mg/ml	30 days
Tobramycin	3 mg/ml	14 mg/ml	30 days
Vancomycin		50 mg/ml	4 days

Anticollagenolytics – serum (α2-macroglobulin antiprotease)
                    – EDTA (chelates Ca^{2+} as enzyme cofactor)
                    – acetyl cysteine (binds Zn^{2+} cofactor)

(Most easily produced by taking autologous blood into EDTA, spinning down and transferring resulting
plasma through several EDTA blood tubes) (Figure 5.9)

Box 5.4 Diagnosis and treatment of collagenolytic 'melting' ulcers

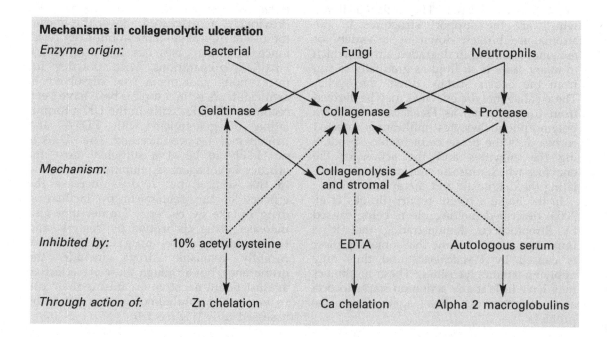

Mechanisms in collagenolytic ulceration

Enzyme origin: Bacterial   Fungi   Neutrophils

                    Gelatinase ← Collagenase → Protease

Mechanism: Collagenolysis
                               and stromal

Inhibited by: 10% acetyl cysteine   EDTA   Autologous serum

Through action of: Zn chelation   Ca chelation   Alpha 2 macroglobulins

Thus, the best therapeutic regimen in the face of a melting ulcer is an aggressive one combining, for the first few hours at least, hourly application of appropriate antibiotic – fortified gentamicin, tobramycin with polymyxin B, or a quinolone such as ciprofloxacin or ofloxacin – with serum containing 0.2M EDTA and an acetylcysteine formulation.

The surgical option of a reasonably deep keratectomy and the placement of a conjunctival pedicle flap should not be overlooked. This will have the advantage of removing a substantial microbial and stromolytic enzyme burden on the one hand, and allowing continual natural application of serum to the ulcerated area through the pedicle flap of conjunctiva.

5.2.7 Chemical injury

Severe corneal ulceration and long-lasting damage to the ocular surface may be caused by chemical injury to the eye. With different chemicals the pathogenesis of damage is very different as is the remedy, although in all cases generous ocular lavage is called for immediately. The centrality of knowing the exact nature of the agent involved shows the importance of taking as thorough a history as possible.

The most serious chemical causing ocular surface damage is alkali – lye or ammonium-based fertilizers are the most commonly encountered alkaline chemicals but burns from such agents are fortunately rare in veterinary ophthalmology. The severity of an alkaline burn stems from the fact that a high pH destroys both epithelium and stroma without causing a coagulative change. In the case of an acid burn, this coagulation prevents further penetration of the chemical and thus limits the depth of the burn. Alkaline burns can be deep and, in addition, they very rapidly destroy all cells in their path, including the stem cells of the corneal epithelium, leading to chronic non-healing ulceration.

Because an alkaline burn acts in many ways like the collagenolysis of a melting ulcer, the same inhibitors of metalloproteinase enzymes are used in addition to copious irrigation of the ocular surface.

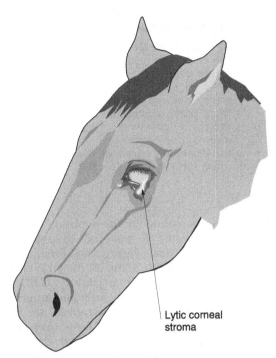

Figure 5.9 Close examination of a wound

Lytic corneal stroma

Controlling the infective agent is important will do little in the short term to prevent stromal degradation by collagenolytic enzymes. We need to inhibit action of these enzymes: difficult, because more than one enzyme is active in most of these ulcers. In fact there is a large family of matrix metallo-proteinases (MMP1–9 at the time of writing) which, together with collagenases and gelatinases, produce the stromolysis. Some of these MMPs are agents of normal corneal remodelling in the healthy eye, while others are derived from infiltrating leucocytes. Still others come from infecting micro-organisms. Each enzyme has a slightly different substrate and a different milieu is required for the inhibition of each one. EDTA binds divalent cations such as Ca^{2+} and since many of these enzymes need calcium as a cofactor, EDTA has an important role in inhibition across the board. Serum alpha 2 macroglobulins similarly are natural inhibitors of a number of these enzymes. Acetylcysteine has an important inhibitory action by chelating zinc.

5.3 Corneoscleral laceration®

5.3.1 Defining the extent of a corneal laceration

Emergency management of a corneal laceration

1. After careful examination, stain eye with fluorescein
2. If non-perforating cover with third eyelid flap or contact lens and treat with atropine and topical antibiotic
3. Definitive repair may involve cyanoacrylate tissue glue or merely contact lens bandaging if superficial and non-perforating
4. If perforating cover with contact lens before definitive repair once oedema has subsided (on atropine and antibiotic treatment topically, with NSAID topically and systemically)
5. Definitive repair in such a case will involve microsurgical repair of corneal laceration

Prognostic indicators in the corneal laceration

1. Substantial corneal oedema and vascularization can resolve after treatment
2. Prolapse of intra-ocular contents (such as iris in a staphyloma) is a poor prognostic sign
3. Length of time between laceration and specialist attention is critical for successful management.

Evaluating the lacerated cornea

- How deep is the laceration?
- Is the laceration perforated? – the Seidel test (see below)
- Are the edges clean or is there foreign material involved?
- Is there other ocular damage?
- Is there one laceration, or several, or a starburst appearance?
- Is the laceration perpendicular to the corneal surface, or with a flap of tissue?

Proper management of a corneoscleral laceration depends on full pre-operative assessment of the degree of injury. It has been found useful in both human and veterinary ophthalmic trauma management to consider this assessment as a hierarchy of injuries and repair techniques. Such a hierarchy begins with the non-perforating corneal laceration. This may be gaping or a self-sealing stromal wound. Next comes the bevelled laceration which, although perforating, has self-closed without involvement of other ocular structures. The more complicated lacerations are those with significant damage to and oedema of surrounding stroma and those in which involvement of iris plugging the leaking wound has created a staphyloma.

Close examination of the wound, ideally with a slit-beam, is essential to evaluate several features (see Figure 5.9). First, how deep is the wound? In some injuries it is clear that the cornea is fully perforated. Others may only involve the epithelium and anterior stroma. The intermediate lacerations are the most difficult to evaluate. There may, for instance, be considerable stromal damage with oedema which may seal a fully perforating wound. The management of a perforating wound is quite different from that of a non-perforating wound, and it is important to define into which category the trauma falls.

The key test here is the Seidel manoeuvre (Figure 5.10). Fluorescein solution 2% is applied to the ocular surface. Even a small amount of aqueous leaving the anterior chamber through a corneal puncture wound will be observed as a clear wandering streak through the fluorescein lake on the ocular surface, leaving no doubt that the cornea is fully perforated. It may be necessary, in the case of a self-closing wound, to perform a forced Seidel test where slight digital pressure is applied to the globe through the upper lid. This presents certain risks and should be done with caution, especially if the corneal stroma appears compromised.

Another important feature is whether the wound gapes at all (Figure 5.11). Some lacerations 'yawn', as it were, at the ocular surface and need a different suturing pattern to ensure correct apposition at the end of surgery. Gaping wounds may be associated with significant anterior and epithelial stromal damage, again requiring different surgical management. Another important feature to note is the amount of corneal

Is there a penetration?

Perform the Seidel Test?

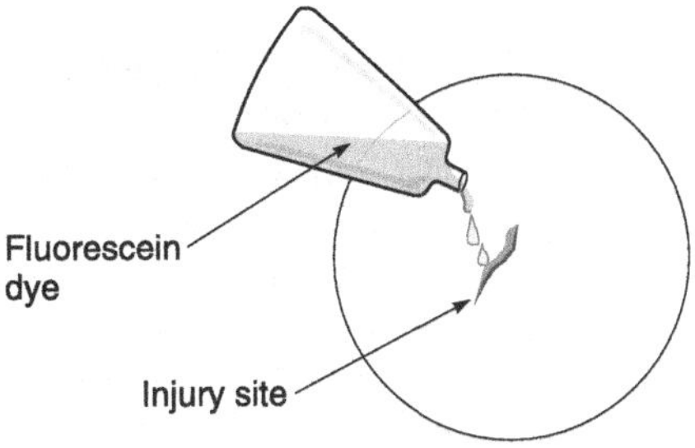

Fluorescein
dye

Injury site

The Seidel Test

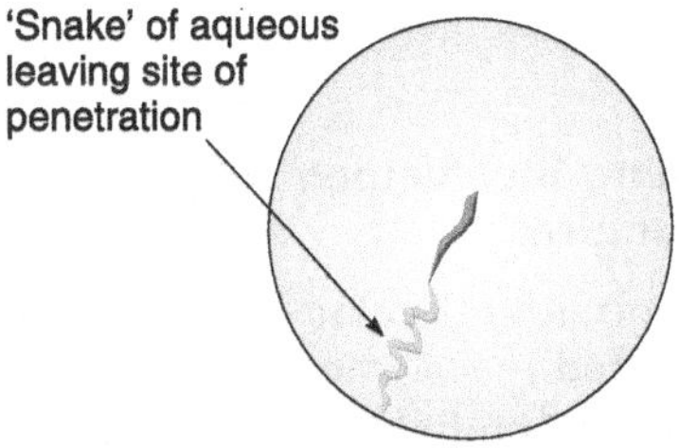

'Snake' of aqueous
leaving site of
penetration

Is there iris prolapse?

Look for dyscoria (abnormal pupil shape)
- Use a stick swab under sterile conditions in
  theatre to remove fibrin/coagulated aqueous
- Assess prolapsed tissue for viability
+ time since prolapse (> or < 24 hours)   <24 hrs } Replace
+ tissue bleeding during manipulation

>24 hrs } excise

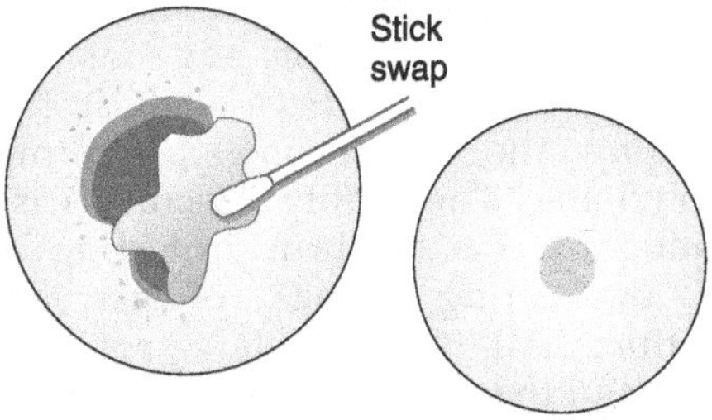

Stick
swap

Figure 5.10 Evaluating a potentially penetrating globe injury

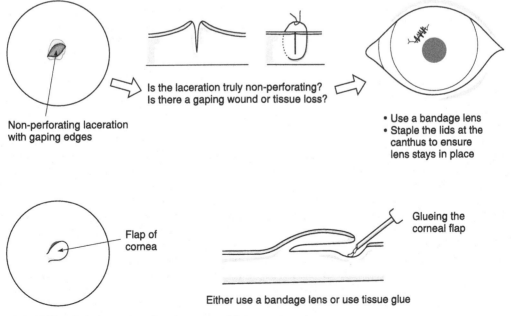

Non-perforating laceration
with gaping edges

Is the laceration truly non-perforating?
Is there a gaping wound or tissue loss?

- Use a bandage lens
- Staple the lids at the
  canthus to ensure
  lens stays in place

Flap of
cornea

Glueing the
corneal flap

Either use a bandage lens or use tissue glue

Figure 5.11 Treating the non-perforating corneal injury

damage surrounding the laceration. This will define where suture entry points can be made, and whether excision of non-viable cornea is needed before the wound edges can be apposed.

5.3.2 Defining involvement of other ocular structures

The most obvious ocular structure which may be affected in a corneal laceration is the iris. The eye is designed, it might be said, to minimize the after-effects of trauma. One of the features of that design is the manner in which the outrush of aqueous after a corneal laceration carries with it the iris, plugging the laceration and forming a staphyloma. The highly vascular iris itself produces a coat of fibrin protecting it from the desiccating effects of its external position. All this renders repair more successful than often appears on first examination of a staphyloma.

Other ocular structures may be involved in a corneal laceration, with or without staphyloma formation. The penetrating agent may have reached the lens surface, where a capsular perforation may result in cataract in the long term or even a so-called phacoanaphylactic reaction upon sudden leakage of lens material.

5.3.3 Repairing a simple non-penetrating corneal laceration

A non-perforating clean laceration, as determined by the Seidel test and in which the edges lie either flat together or gaping open, may be managed appropriately with antibiotic cover and a mild pressure bandage such as that provided by a bandage contact lens. This has the dual effect of supporting the wound by a splinting action and shielding the cornea from the mild abrasion which may occur by natural lid movement. Antibiotic drops such as chloramphenicol or a quinolone should be given two to four times daily. A cycloplegic such as atropine can be useful in preventing ocular pain. After the first day or so it will probably be needed only once daily because of its long duration of action in the otherwise uncompromised eye. If a flap of tissue has been created but not detached from the underlying cornea a thin layer of tissue glue can be painted onto the ulcer bed and the flap replaced (Figure 5.7).

5.3.4 Repairing a simple perforating corneal laceration

Most if not all deep corneal lacerations, and certainly all in which there is still aqueous leakage at the time of examination, require secure wound closure with suture placement. It is important to avoid pressure on the eye during anaesthetic induction or placement of the eyelid speculum. If the globe is already reformed there is no necessity to enter the anterior chamber, but if the chamber needs to be reformed with either balanced salt solution or a visco-elastic this is better irrigated into the anterior chamber through a limbal needle-stab incision rather than through the wound itself, which may be infected or already compromised. When inserting a needle at the limbus it is important to have the needle parallel to the iris, thus not lacerating the iris and causing a haemorrhage from this richly vascularized tissue.

Simple interrupted sutures should be used. The important point is that the sutures should be deep – at least three quarters of the depth of the stroma to ensure that the wound is stable post-surgically (see Figure 5.12). For corneal suturing vicryl or nylon is best; both types of suture are removed when healing is complete. For corneal surgery 6/0 to 10/0 sutures may be used, the thickness being related to availability of microsurgical instruments, means of magnification and surgeon's preference. The sutures should not penetrate the full thickness of the cornea since this gives an excellent wick for entry of infectious organisms from the ocular surface, but a suture that is too shallow results in a gaping wound (see Figure 5.11). The number of sutures should be the minimum required to achieve a watertight closure. Too many sutures result in further stromal compromise. The distance of suture entry from the wound edge is difficult to decide. On the one hand the ideal suture placement is symmetrical, the distance from the wound edge being equal to the depth of the suture. On the other hand the wound edge is often so compromised and oedematous as to render impossible suture entry at the optimal position. In such cases longer sutures can be used but still the intention should be to produce a deep symmetrical

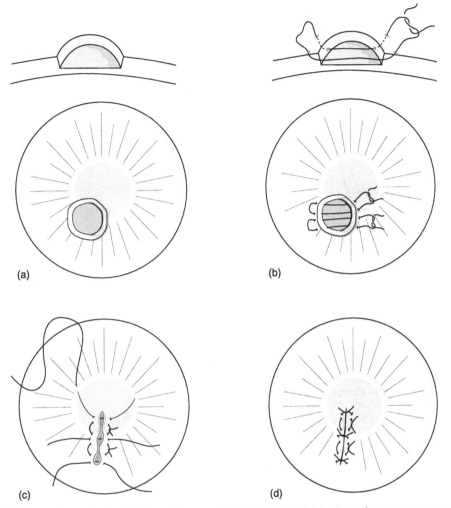

Figure 5.12 Deep ulcer suturing. (a) Frontal/cross-section diagrams; (b) horizontal mattress sutures (small ulcers can be closed with just one horizontal suture; (c) horizontal sutures are slowly drawn tight; (d) initially the cornea is flattened but will return to normal within days

suture. For best suture placement consider the vector forces (Figure 5.11) which render an optimal distance between two interrupted sutures equal to half the distance of the suture-length across the wound (Eisner 1990).

5.3.5 Repairing a corneal laceration complicated by iris inclusion

In a major laceration, or one in which 'shallowing' of the anterior chamber has occurred, iris may be incarcerated in the wound or prolapsed through it (Figure 5.13). In either case iris tissue should be inspected

carefully in deciding whether it should be removed or retained. Incarcerated iris should be freed from the edges of the corneal wound. If the wound is less than 24 hours old it can be replaced in the anterior chamber unless obviously macerated or otherwise damaged. Even after this period healthy-looking tissue can, with care, be replaced. The tissue should also be examined for signs of epithelialization: a grey covering of cells may occur after a day or so. If tissue covered by these cells is replaced, further epithelial cell proliferation may occur giving aberrant epithelialization of anterior segment structures. This can cause

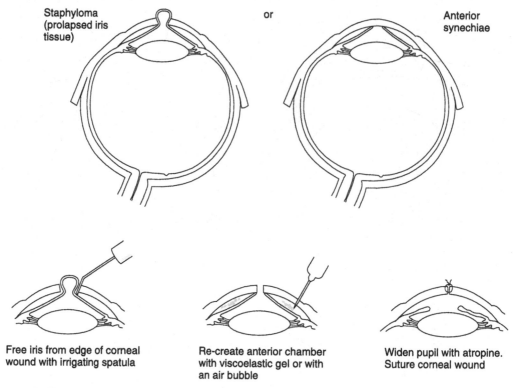

Staphyloma (prolapsed iris tissue)   or   Anterior synechiae

Free iris from edge of corneal wound with irrigating spatula

Re-create anterior chamber with viscoelastic gel or with an air bubble

Widen pupil with atropine. Suture corneal wound

Figure 5.13 Treatment of staphyloma or anterior synechiae

glaucoma if the sheet of growing cells covers the pectinate ligament in the iridocorneal angle.

In the case of prolapsed iridal tissue 24 hours is again an important cut-off point. Before that time dehydration of prolapsed tissue is reduced by the fibrin overlying the prolapsed iris, as discussed above (Figure 5.14). After this time both dehydration from outside, and vascular compromise caused by the iris being entrapped in the corneal wound, tend to cause tissue death in the prolapsed iris.

There are two aims always to be kept in mind: that is, correct reposition of viable iris tissue, as well as adequate closure of the corneal wound. A shallow anterior chamber should first be deepened by the injection of balanced salt solution, or better still visco-elastic, through a paralimbal needle place-ment. Injection through the traumatic wound is more likely to compromise the structures to be manipulated during repositioning and closure. In some cases where the traumatic

wound is presented early, the iridal damage is minimal and iris adhesions to the exposed stroma have yet to occur, repositioning can be by pharmacological means. The pupillary constriction caused by intra-ocular deposition of carbachol or the dilation following intra-cameral 1:10 000 adrenaline may be sufficient to resolve the mild incarceration. More often than not such a regimen is not effective and mechanical repositioning must be attempted. Visco-elastic irrigated into the wound or through a paralimbal paracentesis site may be sufficient to break down early iridostromal adhesions but a more aggressive approach is often needed (see Figure 5.12). The main technique used in such circumstances is one of sweeping the iris off the corneal wound through a paralimbal incision with a cyclo-dialysis spatula or an irrigating cannula. Finally visco-elastic can be deposited to ensure that the iris remains in a posterior position apposed to the lens and not the cornea, or an air bubble can be placed in the anterior chamber as shown opposite.

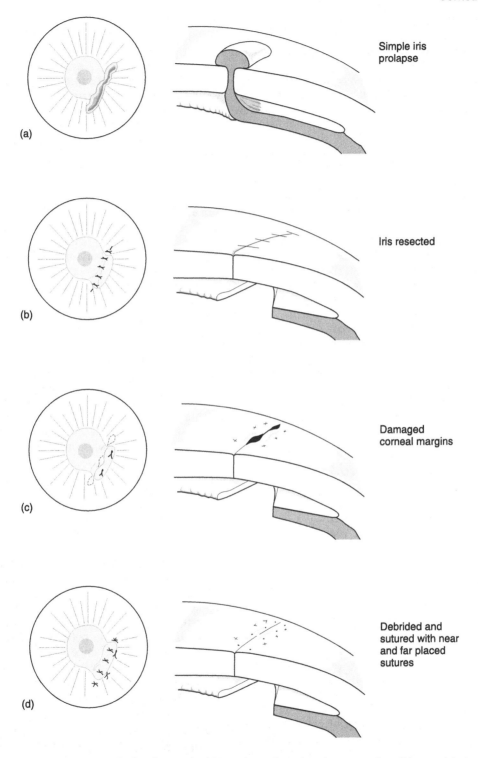

Figure 5.14 Prolapsed iris. (a) Perforating corneal laceration – frontal and cross-section; (b) amputated prolapsed iris, corneal iris adhesions reduced with an iris spatula and suturing of the wound; (c) suturing eyes which present with severe corneal oedema with horizontal sutures should seal the endothelial surface; (d) interrupted sutures placed between the horizontal mattress sutures ensure easy closure of the epithelial edge

The difficult question in these instances is how much iris to excise and how much to reposition. Any iris which has been outside the eye for over 24 hours should be excised and any iridal tissue which does not bleed on handling and starting an excision should be removed. During many such procedures iridal bleeding is encountered. The use of visco-elastic tends to restrict the hyphaema and keep blood localized so as to minimize interference with the surgeon's operating field of view. Again 1:10 000 adrenaline irrigated into the anterior chamber will reduce haemorrhage substantially.

Where lenticular damage has also occurred a decision must be made regarding the advisability of performing lentectomy at the time of primary anterior segment repair. The many problems associated with lentectomy in the face of other post-traumatic ocular complications, such as corneal oedema or iritis, make it unlikely that removal of lens material would be advisable at the time of primary repair. The one situation in which removal of lens material is required early in such ocular trauma management is when capsular rupture leads to the release of lens material into the anterior chamber, when a phacoanaphylactic reaction may occur.

5.4 Corneal foreign body®

5.4.1 Recognizing a corneal foreign body

It might seem easy to identify a corneal foreign body: a piece of plant material, a thorn or a shaft of cat claw should readily be visible in the transparent background of the cornea. Sometimes this is the case. But often significant ocular pathology accompanies the foreign body. Considerable chemosis may obscure the ocular surface or corneal change, such as oedema, infiltration or vascularization, and haemorrhage may complicate the view of a possible foreign body. Often the pain which is associated with a corneal foreign body precludes detailed observation. For all these reasons topical anaesthesia is almost always essential and sedation or brief general anaesthesia may also be necessary.

Several features suggest that a corneal foreign body may be present. Pain is often, but not invariably, a feature. A discharge may be present with corneal pathology such as oedema, infiltration and vascularization. After a traumatic incident giving rise to a corneal foreign body many animals are liable to hide away and not present to the owner for a period, giving time for these sequelae to arise. The problem is that, as well as complicating diagnosis, such signs make it significantly more difficult to remove the foreign body.

If the foreign body is perforating the cornea one may see a uveitis or even a shallow anterior chamber with anterior synechiae or a fibrin clot where there has been leakage. In such cases it is important to refrain from attempting to remove the foreign body until in an aseptic theatre situation with the animal under anaesthetic, so that aqueous leakage through the resulting wound can be dealt with.

In assessing a corneal foreign body it is important to note several features.

1. What is the foreign body? Plant material can be difficult to remove in one piece and may carry potentially dangerous bacteria. It is preferable in such a case not only to culture a bacteriological swab from the trauma site but also to place the material itself on an agar plate and grow organisms directly from it.
2. How deeply is the foreign body penetrating the cornea? A foreign body penetrating the cornea completely but by only a small amount may show few signs of this until it is removed, when aqueous leakage occurs. This is where careful observation from the side as well as in front will allow a better evaluation of depth. Other ocular signs such as mild uveitis, with a slight anisocoria caused by miosis on the affected side, will show that a penetration is likely to have occurred. This is not always the case, since a corneal irritative focus can give rise to a reflex miosis, through a retrograde neural pathway from the trigeminal nerve.

5.4.2 Dealing with a non-perforating corneal foreign body (Figure 5.15)

Removing a foreign body which does not perforate the cornea is clearly a much less hazardous task than dealing with one which

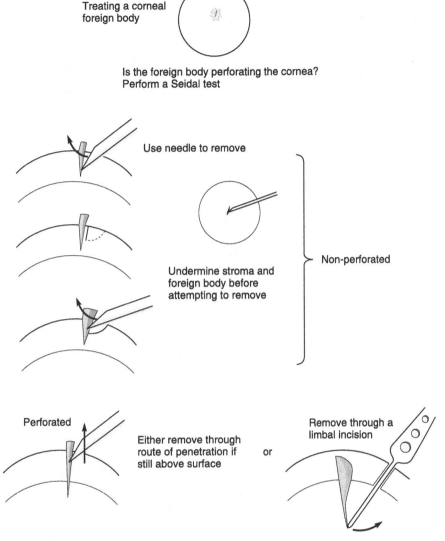

Treating a corneal foreign body

Is the foreign body perforating the cornea?
Perform a Seidal test

Use needle to remove

Undermine stroma and foreign body before attempting to remove

Non-perforated

Perforated

Either remove through route of penetration if still above surface

or

Remove through a limbal incision

Figure 5.15 Treating a corneal foreign body

does penetrate the full thickness of the cornea. Yet the same care should be taken to ensure complete immobility of the patient and good illumination and visibility: without these it is all too easy to worsen the situation or even cause perforation.

The matter is urgent as a foreign body in the cornea for over 24 hours will provoke an inflammatory corneal infiltrate and gradual degradation of surrounding stroma, making removal more difficult. The presence of aqueous flare is common, but more severe anterior segment inflammation and especially a hypopyon should alert one to the possibility of perforation.

First it may be that a very superficial foreign body can be removed simply by irrigation. In any case the ocular surface should be well irrigated and sterilized before an attempt to remove a more deeply lodged foreign body is made. If an initial flushing of the cornea is unsuccessful, as will often be the case, a more interventionist approach should be taken.

The key instrument to be used in removing the majority of foreign bodies is nothing more complicated than a 25 G needle. The most important detail in using the needle is to employ it at 90° to the entry track of the foreign body, as shown in Figure 5.12. In this way one can be sure not to push the item further into the corneal stroma. A moving globe complicates matters considerably, so before removing the foreign body ocular stability must be ensured with haemostats or stay sutures anchoring the conjunctiva at three points. Haemostats can be particularly useful because the one in line with the direction of the entry track can be the fixation against which the foreign body can be withdrawn, as shown in Figure 5.15.

There are times when the foreign body is too deeply embedded to allow a simple removal: where no part of it protrudes beyond the ocular surface. In such cases the easiest method of removal is, using the fine needle and always in the direction by which the foreign body will eventually be removed, to chisel away at the stroma immediately surrounding the surface end of the foreign body, as shown in Figure 5.15. While this will create a small crater leaving a superficial ulcer, it will allow a standard removal of the foreign body by the technique suggested above.

5.4.3 Dealing with a fully penetrating corneal foreign body®

Ensuring globe stasis is even more important where a full perforation of the cornea has occurred. Here we will consider management where the foreign body is still within the body of the stroma and thus is plugging the gap. Larger corneal injuries with involvement of a foreign body are considered under the section on corneal laceration. How is it possible to know, other than by careful clinical examination, that corneal perforation has occurred? If aqueous is leaking from the site of foreign body entry the answer is clear but often the small degree of swelling which accompanies corneal oedema tightly seals the wound, locking the foreign body in place. Then the Seidel test is useful.

With a corneal foreign body that has penetrated the cornea, with some transient loss of aqueous there are four aims to be achieved in dealing with the problem (Figure 5.15). Note that the following list ranks neither these aims in order of importance nor in the order in which they should be remedied.

- First, the foreign body should be removed, maintaining or regaining corneal clarity
- Second, the globe integrity should be maintained, this being particularly important to remember if the corneal deficit after foreign body removal is substantial
- Third, the inflammatory sequelae of loss of aqueous must be remedied or hopefully prevented
- Fourth, intra-ocular or corneal stromal infection should similarly be remedied or prevented.

The last two of these should be considered first when dealing with a lacerated cornea. Antibiotic and anti-inflammatory treatment should be in place before attempting surgically to correct the damage present as a consequence of a penetrating foreign body. Intensive topical and systemic antibiosis is critical given the likelihood that microbial contamination will occur either in the corneal stroma or the anterior segment. Choosing the antibiotic to use has been covered above but it is important to repeat that the involvement of plant material as the foreign body must always alert one to the possibility of fungal infection.

With any corneal perforation inflammatory sequelae can cause significant morbidity in the eye. In the case of a penetrating foreign body there may be considerable loss of aqueous as the foreign body is removed. In this situation both the loss and its prostaglandin-mediated inflammatory consequences can be controlled. Where relatively little loss has occurred with a penetrating foreign body, there is ample opportunity to give a topical non-steroidal anti-inflammatory agent such as flurbiprofen (Ocufen), diclofenac (Voltarol) or ketorolac (Acular) before attempting surgical removal. Where aqueous loss has already happened, as in a corneal laceration, any ameliorative anti-inflammatory action is rather late. However, surgical intervention will cause further fluid loss and inhibiting the prostaglandin-mediated inflammatory response as above is still important.

After these partially reparative and partially prophylactic steps have been taken, the foreign body can be removed. The important feature of such a removal, as with that of a non-penetrating foreign body, is not to make matters worse. It is so tempting to use a small pair of forceps and try to pluck the foreign body from the corneal surface. Too often, however, this merely results in embedding the item further in the stroma or, worse still, pushing it through into the anterior chamber. Here it floats and is significantly more difficult to apprehend and remove from the eye.

A foreign body embedded in and perforating the depth of the stroma can be carefully removed with a needle as for the non-perforating foreign body. It may be necessary to enlarge the entry wound with a needle or blade, having already stabilized the foreign body to ensure it is not lost into the anterior chamber. The most difficult cases are those in which the majority of the foreign body has passed into the anterior chamber leaving a small stub in the posterior stroma. In such a case removal should not be retrograde, reversing the entry path of the foreign body through the cornea, but further through the anterior chamber using microforceps through a limbal incision (Figure 5.15).

5.5 Antibiosis and mydriatic cycloplegia in corneal emergencies

The reader is referred to the opening chapter of this volume for a fuller discussion of the diagnosis and treatment of infectious ocular disease. Again we emphasize the benefits of taking samples and using in the first place a broad-spectrum antibiotic. The samples can be examined directly after appropriate staining with Gram's method, Giemsa or Diff Quik techniques and with lactophenol cotton blue for fungal hyphal elements as well as for bacteriological and fungal culture.

With regard to analgesia, paralysis of the ciliary body is a useful analgesic adjunct in iritis, as above. This also applies in corneal disease where miosis is noted, the iridal spasm being caused by retrograde trigeminal nerve conduction. In every corneal condition presenting with apparent pain or a degree of anisocoria, a mydriatic cycloplegic agent should be used.

Chapter 6

Iris

6.1 Iritis®

Iritis is one of the key conditions causing the red eye. It can be painful and sight-threatening and thus is an important condition calling

Emergency management of anterior uveitis

1. Perform full ophthalmic examination
2. Measure intra-ocular pressure
3. Evaluate possibility of systemic infection (Gram-negative bacteria, *Toxoplasma*, viral disease)
4. Treat with mydriatic until mydriasis is achieved
5. Treat with topical steroid if no corneal ulceration present, otherwise use topical non-steroidal agent
6. Treat with systemic steroid if severe or non-responsive to topical steroid alone
7. Refer for treatment with tissue plasminogen activating factor if substantial fibrin deposition occurs

Prognostic indicators in anterior uveitis

1. Substantial intra-ocular haemorrhage a poor prognostic sign
2. Substantial posterior synechiae non-responsive to mydriasis a poor prognostic sign
3. Concurrent posterior segment signs such as retinal detachment a poor prognostic sign
4. Viral systemic cause a poor prognostic sign for the uveitis and the systemic health of the animal

for immediate and sustained action. Inflammation of the iris is a relatively common condition in small animal ophthalmology. It forms the most obvious part of uveitis, inflammation of the uveal tract which also comprises the ciliary body and the choroid. While intermediate and posterior uveitis causing inflammation of the ciliary body or choroid are not noticed by the owner they can provide useful signs to the veterinary surgeon investigating a uveitic eye.

6.1.1 Diagnosis: clinical signs

The classic signs of an anterior uveitis are related to anterior uveal inflammation, iridal muscle spasm and, in many cases, ciliary body dysfunction (Figure 6.1). The key features of inflammation have always been defined as *rubor, calor, tumor et dolor* together with reduction of function.

Rubor, redness, is seen in iritis in the increased vasculature of rubeosis iridis. Iridal vasculature is in some places dilated and in other constricted. Where vascular dilation occurs the iris appears criss-crossed with engorged vessels giving a rubeotic appearance, hence the term rubeosis iridis. In areas of vascular constriction ischaemia occurs. Ischaemic tissue releases angiogenic factors which promote new blood vessel formation seen as small vascular sprouts in rubeosis iridis. Redness is also manifest in the episclera as the red eye and is due to vascular dilation secondary to inflammatory cytokine production.

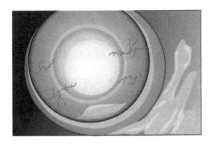

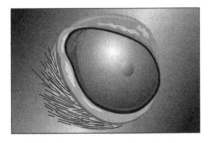

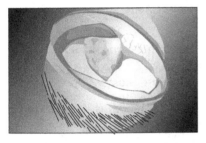

Figure 6.1 The classic signs of an anterior uveitis are related to anterior uveal inflammation, iridal muscle spasm and, in many cases, ciliary body dysfunction giving reduced intraocular pressure

Calor, heat, is difficult to determine in the eye. *Tumor*, swelling, is seen in the swollen dull-coloured iris. In some cases, especially with a lightly pigmented iris, the formation of raised lymphoid follicles within the iris tissue can be visualized, especially with a slit lamp or slit setting in a direct ophthalmoscope which readily demonstrates a raised profile.

Dolor, pain, is a frequently presenting sign in uveitis. It is predominantly related to iridal and ciliary body muscular spasm. Photophobia is also a classical sign, although exactly where the mechanism of photophobia lies is still unclear: it may be related to muscular spasm as the pupillary light reflex occurs. Knowing the mechanism of pain generation is at the heart of ocular analgesia,

is very important and is discussed in section 6.1.3.

The glory of the eye and of ophthalmology is that tissue changes can be directly assessed by ophthalmoscopy. This is particularly true in uveitis. Early influx of leucocytes into the iris and the formation of lymphoid follicles are often visible even at the very earliest stages. Thickening of the iris and loss of iris surface detail are other results of cellular infiltration into the body of the iris. Leucocyte diapedesis from the iris surface, and fibrin formation and release from iridal and ciliary body vasculature result in flare. In flare, particles such as cells and fibrin form a haze in the anterior chamber through the Tyndall effect when a beam of light is shone through the anterior chamber. With experience flare can be graded, allowing a semi-quantitative estimate of the degree of inflammation. While this is not particularly useful in comparing disease in different animals, it plays an important part in determining whether uveitis is improving under treatment.

A higher number of cells in the aqueous results in deposit of cells on the posterior face of the cornea as keratic precipitates. These may have different appearances depending on the type of cells and the inflammatory processes involved. Non-granulomatous inflammation may show small keratic precipitates with a wide distribution across the cornea. Granulomatous inflammation produces larger keratic precipitates, often known as mutton fat KPs. These may form a crescent in the inferior cornea Cells fall in the downward current, as cooler aqueous falls in the centre of the anterior chamber and then rises at the limbus. The bicircular aqueous currents thus formed are slowest at the lowest point where they change direction (Figure 6.1) and the cells are thus deposited in this position. If a larger number of cells enter the aqueous they fall under gravity to give a hypopyon in the ventral anterior chamber. Thus, the degree of anterior segment inflammatory change can readily be assessed by visualizing cell infiltration directly.

Posterior segment inflammation is important in investigations also. The uvea, as detailed above, comprises the iris, the ciliary body and the choroid. Fundoscopy of the uveitic eye may show anterior vitreal cell-related flare in pars planitis (intermediate uveitis), or chorioretinal inflammatory exudate or retinal detachment in posterior uveitis. Where there is an anterior uveitis in one eye but on casual examination an apparently normal fellow eye, it is always worth performing fundoscopy on both eyes even if this means waiting some time for mydriasis to take effect. Finding signs of a posterior uveitis in the other eye will make the difference between topical therapy in the unilateral anterior inflammation and systemic anti-inflammatory medication in the bilateral panuveitis.

Iridal muscle spasm manifests as pupil constriction, miosis. This, combined with the readiness of the pupil to adhere to the underlying lens, produces posterior synechiae which can, in an untreated eye, result in a permanently miotic pupil or iris bombé. In the latter case iridal adhesion to the lens prevents movement of aqueous forward through the pupil and hence gives a precipitous increase in intra-ocular pressure. All these possibilities render amelioration of miosis an exceptionally important factor in treatment of the uveitic eye, as discussed in section 6.1.5.

It may seem that the ciliary body, being invisible by routine fundoscopy, has few secrets to give away in the investigation of the uveitic eye. Yet when we consider reduction in function as a key feature of inflammation, the ciliary body gives the only quantifiable feature in uveitis: the level of intra-ocular pressure. While it may be thought that the diagnosis of glaucoma is the only reason for the measurement of intra-ocular pressure, determination of pressure in the uveitic eye should perhaps be considered equally important. A uveitic eye with a low intra-ocular pressure has an active uveal inflammation, while a treated eye with a higher (but still abnormally low) pressure than at the previous examination, is an eye with a resolving uveitis. Tonometry is thus a key diagnostic step in uveitis.

6.1.2 Diagnosis: diagnostic tests

It might be thought that the clinical appearance of a uveitic eye is sufficient foundation on which to base a diagnosis of uveitis. Clinical signs together with a measurement of a low intra-ocular pressure are indeed sufficient

Emergency management of hyphaema

1. Perform full ophthalmic examination, noting concurrent signs of uveitis or glaucoma
2. Measure intra-ocular pressure and treat accordingly if raised
3. Perform ocular ultrasonography if available, looking for tissue trauma or intra-ocular tumour
4. If recurring hyphaema without signs of ocular trauma, evaluate dog for haemorrhage elsewhere and perform coagulation profile
5. Give topical steroids if ulceration is not present and signs of uveitis are present
6. Give topical NSAIDs if ulceration is present
7. Give topical atropine if uveitis is present but not if glaucoma supervenes
8. Tissue plasminogen activating factor may be useful in resolving a clot, but care is needed as this can cause further haemorrhage

Prognostic indicators in hyphaema

1. Signs of intra-ocular neoplasia are clearly a poor prognostic sign
2. Supervening glaucoma and the darkening of the blood as it clots are poor prognostic signs
3. Recurring hyphaema may signal a systemic coagulopathy or intra-ocular structural defect involving vasculature, both of which are poor prognostic signs

Differential diagnosis in hyphaema

- Ocular trauma
- Uveitis
- Intra-ocular tumour
- Coagulopathy
- Retinal detachment (in more chronic detachments)
- Retinal vascular haemorrhage (such as occurs in Collie Eye Anomaly)

Thus work up for hyphaema should include:
Further ocular examination (signs of uveitis, lesions in fellow eye)
Ocular ultrasound (retinal detachment, intra-ocular tumour)
Coagulopathy work up (platelet count, clotting time, PPT, APT)

as a basis but confirmation can be gained by performing a paracentesis. A cytocentrifugation of 0.2 ml of aqueous will show the cell types and indicate whether any infection is present by documenting local antibody production. This might be seen as somewhat academic, but the important diagnostic tests, especially in cats, are those which determine whether a viral aetiology underlies the uveitis. Serology for FIP, FeLV, FIP and *Toxoplasma* is considered the standard systemic work up routine in Britain. Note that with travel of animals abroad increasing recently Leishmania and Ehrlichia should be included as differentials for uveitis. In the USA serology should be carried out for fungal agents such as *Blastomyces* and *Coccidioides,* which cause systemic fungal disease not infrequently manifesting as ocular disease. *Bartonella henslae* is another organism recently found associated with feline uveitis. In all these cases determining the ratio of aqueous to serum antibody titre is vastly superior to serology alone (Chauvkin et al. 1994).

A different set of pathogens may be important in equine recurrent uveitis: *Leptospira* species and particularly *L. interrogans* have been found in a significant proportion of cases while *Brucella, Toxoplasma* and possibly equine herpes virus 1 may be involved. Documenting which organism is involved is probably not particularly important, although treatment of toxoplasmosis with a drug such as clindamycin may be valuable in addition to the classical topical anti-inflammatories.

6.1.3 Treatment: pain relief

As has been noted above, pain relief in uveitis should be an admixture of spasmolytic analgesia through cycloplegia, analgesia through the anti-inflammatory action of the non-steroidal agents and in addition classical analgesia with opiates if necessary. Early reduction of ciliary body spasm and early anti-inflammatory medication reduce pain quite substantially without resort to the more powerful systemic analgesics.

6.1.4 Treatment: anti-inflammatory medication

Since inflammatory disease is at the heart of uveitis, anti-inflammatory medication must be at the centre of anti-uveitic therapy. Such treatment needs to be titrated relative to the severity of the uveitis and its position. A mild anterior uveitis will require topical 1% prednisolone acetate. A severe uveitis with posterior segment involvement will require systemic (per os) predisolone at the anti-inflammatory dose of 1.5 mg/kg or even azathioprine.

Subconjunctival injection in an already painful eye can be eased dramatically by the application of topical anaesthetic. Merely placing a drop of proxymetacaine or amethocaine in the eye will, however, have a limited effect. A much more effective protocol is to soak a cotton-tipped swab in the anaesthetic and press it onto the globe in the position where the injection will be given. This produces profound local anaesthesia in a focused area not just superficially on the conjunctiva but deep in the episclera and sclera.

6.1.5 Treatment: reducing miosis and preventing synechia formation

One of the key concepts to bear in mind when faced with an emergency is that the first time the patient is seen is the best (and sometimes the only) opportunity to reduce disease activity and signs. This is certainly the case with the profound miosis seen in acute uveitis and the formation of synechiae so common in intra-ocular inflammation.

A uveitic eye with a miotic pupil needs attention until the pupil is dilated, not a quick application of atropine and re-examination in a few days time. Often atropine is sufficient to produce mydriasis in a mild uveitis, but even in such a case the response to a long-acting mydriatic such as atropine is difficult to gauge at the first consultation. A first application of mydriatic should include tropicamide as well as atropine to ensure rapid mydriasis. Should both of these fail, phenylephrine can be added and the three drugs used together every 15 minutes until mydriasis is achieved. Should all topical mydriatics fail to act adequately, a subconjunctival injection of 0.05 ml 1% atropine, 0.05 ml 1% tropicamide and 0.05 ml 10% phenylephrine should be given. There is some risk of a systemic reaction and cardiovascular parameters should be monitored immediately before and

Pathogenic mechanisms in uveitis

- Inflammatory cell infiltration   lymphoid nodules in iris stroma
  inflammatory cells in keratic
  precipitates larger number of cells form hypopyon

- Iris ischaemia   from vessel constriction giving rise to new vessel sprouts
  (rubeosis iridis)

- Pupillary constriction   through muscular spasm producng miosis

- Iridal adhesion   posterior synechiae (iris-lens adhesion) and also peripheral
  anterior synechiae which can lead to glaucoma

- Pain   particularly through ciliary body spasm also because of
  photophobia (mechanism unclear)

Thus treatment must   **reduce inflammation** (steroid and NSAIDs)

reduce pain (analgesics but also cycloplegics to reduce
ciliary spasm)

dilate pupil (mydriatic high dose frequency)

after such a subconjunctival injection. There is evidence that reduction of inflammation will promote the action of topical mydriatics. Thus, should mydriasis not occur it is worth hospitalizing the animal and trying again after a few hours of intensive anti-inflammatory medication.

At this point it is important to note that use of powerful agents such as atropine in horses must be approached with caution. The possibility of development of ileus even with topical use of atropine must always be remembered and use of an atropine ointment, with concomitant reduction of systemic absorption, is to be recommended.

Another peculiarity of the equine eye is the recent use of vitrectomy to treat recurrent cases of uveitis (Frühauf et al. 1998). The removal of pathogens such as *Leptospira* may be important, or it may be the removal of the 'soup' of inflammatory mediators which remain in the vitreous which is important. Nevertheless vitrectomy can certainly be useful in reducing the frequency and severity of attacks in horses. It may be that in the future this approach will show benefit in the dog and cat also, where recurrent or persistent intra-ocular inflammation is a significant problem.

6.2 Change in iris appearance

Clearly a case of iritis, as discussed above, will cause changes in iris appearance: new vascularization, iris swelling, miosis and iridal darkening all cause such changes. There are other lesions which alter iris appearance: neoplasia is one. Iris masses may be primary tumours, part of a more generalized disease such as feline lymphosarcoma complex or a sign of metastolic disease from a tumour elsewhere.

The development of benign iris pigmentation is another which may be rapidly developing and therefore a potential neoplasm requiring immediate intervention. The differential diagnosis of a benign iris pigmentary naevus and a diffuse iris melanoma can be difficult, particularly in the cat (Williams 1994). In some cases the raised profile of an iris melanoma above the iris is pathognomonic but in other animals diffuse iris melanoma and iris naevi can appear identical. One might think that the naevi would be congenital and not change in appearance from birth. Yet in the authors' experience feline iris pigmentation can develop rapidly and in a multifocal manner which is indistinguishable from melanoma. Given the poor prognosis of feline iris melanoma once it reaches the iridal periphery and associated limbal and ciliary body vasculature, enucleation is the preferred option.

The key factor here, as in any veterinary medicine, is without a doubt client communication. In such a case the outcome can always seem negative. If the lesion is neoplastic the cat has a chance of systemic metastasis. If the lesion is benign the eye will have been removed to no purpose. If the client is informed that the condition may be benign, but that the eye should be removed in case a neoplasm is present, then the outcome can always be presented as positive: either the lesion was neoplastic but we have removed it early and therefore the prognosis is good; or the lesion was benign so no neoplasm was present, the cat will live a normal, if unocular, life and the client can be reassured that tumour was not present.

It may seem strange to include this section in a book on emergency ophthalmology. Yet in the emergency consultation optimal client communication is supremely important. The very fact that the animal has been presented as an emergency shows that owner is worried by an acute problem. It is at this very point that the veterinarian's calm well-informed manner reassures the owner and ensures that the animal benefits through the strengthening of the client–veterinarian relationship.

Chapter 7

Glaucoma

7.1 Introductory remarks

Glaucoma is a condition of increased intra-ocular pressure that may be seen in patients secondary to intra-ocular inflammation, intra-ocular neoplasia or more often in the dog as a progressive disease resulting from inherited abnormality of the irido-corneal angle (Figure 7.1).

A large number of dog breeds have been shown to have an inherited dysplasia of structures in the iridocorneal angle (ACVO 1996, Whitley et al. 1995) shown in Table 7.1. Several features of glaucoma are particularly important in an emergency situation but the main problem with glaucoma is the long-term control of intra-ocular pressure either by ocular medication or by surgery.

Glaucoma is a blinding, painful condition and in many cases the changes which cause pain and result in blindness occur in the first few hours of an acute episode of glaucoma and need rapid treatment to reduce the intra-ocular pressure.

The key diagnostic aid in glaucoma is measurement of intra-ocular pressure. As we have noted earlier, having a tonometer to

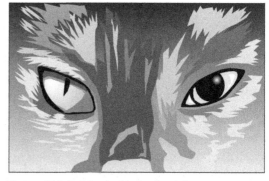

Figure 7.1 Is this uveitis in the right eye or glaucoma in the left?

Table 7.1 Dog breeds predisposed to glaucoma

Akita	Chihuahua	Lakeland terrier	Sealyham terrier
Alaskan malaute	Dalmatian	Maltese	Shih tzu
American cocker spaniel	Dandie dinmont terrier	Miniature pinscher	Siberian husky
Basset hound	Daschund	Miniature schnauzer	Skye terrier
Beagle	English cocker spaniel	Norfolk terrier	Smooth fox terrier
Border collie	German shepherd	Norwegian elkhound	Tibetan terrier
Boston terrier	Giant schnauzer	Norwich terrier	Welsh springer spaniel
Bouvier de Flandres	Greyhound	Poodle	Welsh terrier
Brittany spaniel	Irish setter	Samoyed	West Highland White terrier
Cairn terrier	Italian greyhound	Scottish terrier	Wire fox terrier
Cardigan Welsh corgi			

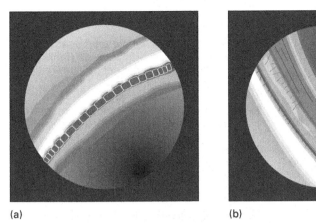

(a)   (b)

Figure 7.2 Normal (a) and abnormal (b) iridocorneal angle

hand is important and acquiring and regularly using a Schiotz tonometer, as described in Appendix A, is highly recommended.

The long-term control of intra-ocular pressure should be undertaken by referral to a veterinary ophthalmologist.

An important aspect of glaucoma presenting unilaterally is the possible future involvement of the remaining visual eye. Several studies have shown that topical anti-glaucoma treatment of the non-glaucomatous eye can prevent or at least postpone the disease in this eye.

7.2. Diagnosis

7.2.1 Clinical signs

The eye with acute glaucoma is, together with globe prolapse, one of the few extreme ocular emergencies. In the vast majority of cases the eye is red and painful and immediate reduction in ocular pressure is required to ameliorate these signs. More important in the long term is the effect of high intra-ocular pressure on vision. The acutely glaucomatous eye is blind and, without a rapid reduction in intra-ocular pressure, this loss of vision will be permanent.

7.2.2 Diagnostic tests

The key diagnostic test in glaucoma as we recognize it in veterinary ophthalmology is measurement of intra-ocular pressure (IOP). In human ophthalmology, while glaucoma used to be defined as ocular disease associated with increased IOP, the tendency recently has been to move away from IOP as the defining criterion of glaucoma. Some eyes with a raised IOP have no signs of ocular disease nor visual defect (Figure 7.2). In these cases people are said to have ocular hypertension but not glaucoma. Conversely there are a growing number of people with loss of visual fields as determined by perimetry and a cupped optic disc, the classic signs of glaucoma, but with a normal or even low intra-ocular pressure (Figure 7.3). These cases are termed 'low tension glaucoma', a description which used to be considered an

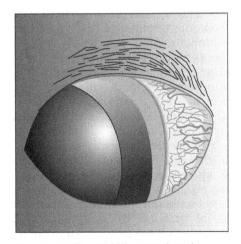

Figure 7.3 Closed iridocorneal angle

oxymoron. It may be wondered what relevance this has to the veterinary field. The importance is that glaucoma is now recognized as a disease with its origin not primarily in the iridocorneal angle, where all the attention used to be focused, but in the optic disc. The optic neuropathy in classical glaucoma is related to and indeed directly caused by increased IOP. But optic nerve changes may be caused by degenerative or vascular changes in the nerve head as well as by the physical damage associated with increased IOP. It is not being suggested that we should forget high IOP as the predominant cause of glaucoma in animals, but rather that we should broaden our view regarding the mechanisms underlying sight loss in the disease. Currently this may have little impact on how we treat glaucoma in our patients, which are generally so much more advanced in ocular deterioration than are human patients who present with early glaucoma. But in the future new agents may be introduced adding to the small armamentarium of anti-glaucoma drugs we possess at present.

Emergency management of glaucoma

1. Perform full ophthalmic examination
2. Determine cause of glaucoma (inherited with gonioscopic changes, post-uveitis, lens luxation etc.)
3. Measure intra-ocular pressure
4. If IOP over 30 mmHg give 20% mannitol solution intravenously at 1–2 g/kg over 30 minutes
5. Start topical carbonic anhydrase inhibitor treatment at least q.i.d.
6. Monitor intra-ocular pressure hourly in acute phase

Prognostic indicators in glaucoma

1. Degree and duration of intra-ocular pressure increase are critical in prognosis
2. Degree of visual loss in eye important
3. Presence of optic disc cupping a poor prognostic sign
4. History of previous ocular signs or disease in other eye generally a poor prognostic sign

---

7.3 Treatment

7.3.1 Immediate systemic hypotensive therapy®

Treatment in the emergency situation where a dog presents with a high IOP in primary glaucoma is, and has been for many years, the use of systemic hyperosmotic agents. Intravenous mannitol at up to 2 g/kg or oral glycerol at 2 ml/kg acts to draw fluid from both the anterior segment of the eye and the vitreous humour. They act rapidly and for several hours reduce intra-ocular pressure by 10+ mmHg, reducing a pathologically high pressure to normality. In an emergency situation where no such agents are available or where a systemic condition such as renal disease precludes use of a hyperosmotic agent, a 25 G needle can gently be driven at an angle through the sclera at the limbus, allowing aqueous just to fill the needle hub before the needle is withdrawn. Such a procedure is not without complications: the rapid reduction of pressure by such a physical method may result in intra-ocular bleeding and is probably only to be recommended when performed by an ophthalmologist with expertise in emergency management of glaucoma. Systemic osmotic agents also have their disadvantages, particularly contra-indication in cases of renal failure. Since they are to be used in the emergency situation, little time is available for a full renal work up. Nevertheless a careful history will ascertain whether the animal is polydipsic and therefore likely to have renal compromise. A rapid evaluation of blood urea can be performed in order more fully to ensure that one is not going to save the eye while ignoring the more general problems of the animal.

7.3.2 Long-term reduction of IOP®

The problem with a stabilized acute glaucoma is what to do to maintain low pressure in a glaucomatous eye in the face of abnormally low aqueous drainage. This question presents itself soon after stabilization with oral or intravenous osmotic ocular hypotensive drugs as discussed above, as it is not advisable to give more than two administrations of mannitol or glycerol to any one animal.

Detailed discussion of methods of long-term management of glaucoma might seem inappropriate here, as they are not aimed at the emergency situation. Briefly, the optimal long-term management is surgical. While long-term medical inhibition of aqueous production is possible, since the withdrawal of dichlorphenamide from the market no one drug is particularly efficacious. Nevertheless Trusopt, a topical CAI, can be useful for control of mild glaucoma.

More invasive methods to reduce aqueous production involve ciliary body ablation, either by trans-scleral photo-ablation using a laser or by trans-scleral cryosurgery. While these carry a risk of severe damage to other ocular structures and associated intra-ocular inflammatory sequelae, they have been used with success in sighted eyes. Intravitreal genticin has been used successfully pharmacologically to ablate the ciliary body but should be reserved for blind painful eyes (but probably not in cats, for fear of causing posterior segment post-traumatic sarcoma). This treatment is not advised in the emergency situation and the reader is referred to published reports for further information.

Pharmacological reduction of aqueous formation by carbonic anhydrase inhibition

has been achieved with dichlorphenamide (Daranide) for many years, but now that this drug has been withdrawn in favour of the topical dorzolamide (Trusopt) other agents will have to be employed by those not favouring a surgical treatment. Acetazolamide (Diamox) is another carbonic anhydrase inhibitor but works less well than dichlorphenamide and tends to have worse emetic and nauseous side effects. Methazolamide (Naptazane) has not, to our knowledge, been assessed in dogs.

Other drugs regularly used in human glaucoma relax the musculature of the ciliary body. In the primate eye at least these have a major effect on the outflow capacity of the drainage pathways. Whether this is the case in the dog is rather unclear because dogs do not accommodate to a great extent. Their ciliary musculature is therefore not particularly well-developed and relaxing ciliary muscle in non-primate mammals has less effect on the drainage pathways. This means that many of the drugs used in people have questionable efficacy in dogs.

Nevertheless cholinergic miotics are useful in the dog. They probably act in a more complex way in the dog than in man, widening the sclerociliary cleft by a compound action involving the iris sphincter muscle as well as the ciliary body musculature. Certainly demecarium bromide (Humorsol), a long-acting anticholinesterase, works extremely well but is only available in the United States. Pilocarpine, a direct-acting parasympathomimetic, is perhaps the most commonly used miotic. A single dose reduces intra-ocular pressure for six to eight hours; 4% drops produce no greater pressure reduction than do 2% drops, but a gel formulation gives longer-lasting pressure reduction, at least in people.

Other ocular hypotensive preparations which could potentially be used in the dog include adrenergic agonists acting on both alpha and beta receptors. Topical alpha agonists, such as apraclonidine, cause vasoconstriction of vessels in the ciliary processes thus decreasing aqueous humour production. But they also dilate the pupil, with pressure-increasing effects in man but less so in the dog. Beta receptor effects of adrenergic agonists increase aqueous production but also act directly on the trabecular meshwork to increase outflow. Thus an agent such as epinephrine, or the less irritant pro-drug dipivalyl epinephrine, variously increases and decreases pressure through actions on alpha and beta receptors. In man, and in the dog, the overall effect is to lower pressure. The complicating factor is that beta antagonists as well as agonists have pressure-lowering effects. Beta blocking agents bind to receptors in the ciliary epithelium and reduce aqueous secretion. In human ophthalmology, timolol maleate has a major role as a topical antiglaucoma drug. Timolol has no effects on the pupil, accommodation or outflow facility but can reduce aqueous production in man by nearly 50% at concentrations as low as 0.25%. In the dog, concentrations up to 20 times that amount are required to give significant reductions in intraocular pressure (Gelatt 4% paper).

To return to the question regarding whether glaucoma pathology is at the iridocorneal angle, where so many of these drugs act, or at the optic nerve head, it is now being suggested that perhaps the beta blockers have more effect on the vasculature around the optic nerve head than they do on the iridocorneal angle or the ciliary body. Indeed there are other workers who claim that by reducing aqueous production with medication these drugs are starving the iridocorneal angle cells of the nutritious aqueous they need to survive – possibly iridocorneal angle pathology is being made worse!

7.3.3 Neuroprotection

As noted above a recent change of emphasis has occurred in glaucoma pathophysiology. The focus on ocular damage from merely high intra-ocular pressure caused by impaired iridocorneal angle drainage has moved to effects of pressure and other factors on the optic nerve head and its vasculature.

We have known for many years that disc cupping leads to visual impairment. An extension of that concept leads to the hypothesis that blindness in glaucoma is predominantly related to optic nerve pathology. Does this change of emphasis change our treatment regimens for glaucoma patients? In one sense it changes nothing. For the vast majority of canine and feline glaucoma patients the problem is high intraocular pressure and the necessary treatment lowers that pressure. But in another sense it changes a lot. If optic nerve damage is the focus of glaucoma pathology then at least part of our glaucoma therapy should be aimed at neuroprotection.

The sort of tissue changes and mechanisms at the heart of optic nerve damage relate to events such as calcium influx to nerve cells after damage. Any neural damage, be it related to a head injury, a cerebrovascular accident or pressure-induced damage of ganglion cell axons in the optic nerve head, produces a chain reaction of neurotransmitter-related events resulting in the opening of neural ion channels which allow the lethal influx of calcium ions into neurons. If this can be prevented, perhaps by the use of calcium channel blockers such as verapamil, some of the long-term damage associated with the sudden rise in IOP in acute glaucoma (seen so often in dogs with compromised iridocorneal angle aqueous drainage) may also be prevented.

This, however, is all in the future – the key factors in diagnosing and treating glaucoma in the emergency situation are being able to recognize the signs, confirm the diagnosis by tonometry and then lower the pressure with systemic osmotic ocular hypotensive agents before deciding what to do for the long-term improvement of aqueous drainage in such cases.

Chapter 8

Lens

Conditions of the lens presenting as emergencies are luxation and damage. Much regarding this latter situation is covered above as a complication of globe perforation but here the consequences of lens rupture will be noted. The only other acute condition of the lens which could present as an emergency is a rapidly progressing cataract, such as is seen in diabetes. This also is discussed here, although the diagnosis is normally easy and management is cataract extraction. Sudden onset cataract might not be covered as an emergency in some texts. It is sufficiently concerning for owners to be presented as an emergency and therefore is covered here.

8.1 Lens luxation®

The clearest emergency presenting as a disease of the lens is lens luxation. Once seen never forgotten: lens luxation is obvious in its presentation once one knows what to look for. The characteristics of the animal involved can be very instructive This condition often occurs in middle-aged terrier breeds and sudden ocular pain or discomfort in such a dog should focus one's attention on lens luxation as a likely diagnosis. The ocular signs can be immediately diagnostic. There is a red eye with raised pressure and an aphakic crescent where the lens is obviously displaced from its normal central position, leaving an area where an uninterrupted tapetal reflex can be seen between lens and pupillary margin (Figure 8.1). If there are also lens changes such as cataract the edge of the lens can be seen even more clearly and the diagnosis be made.

In other cases the lens luxates completely into the anterior chamber. Here it may be possible to see reflected light beautifully outlining the lens (Figure 8.2). In such a case an area of corneal oedema often occurs where the lens presses on the corneal endothelium.

Unfortunately, diagnosis is not so easy in many cases. Lens luxation may occur anteriorly followed by a falling back of the lens behind the iris and diagnosis can be difficult if an aphakic crescent is not obvious. Since the iris is not supported by the lens posteriorly in such cases it wobbles on slight manipulation of the head. As 'iris wobble' sounds less than 100% scientific, the term iridodonesis is used.

Signs of lens luxation are

- Lens clearly present in anterior chamber
- Lens clearly eccentric in position with an aphakic crescent visible
- Lens less obviously displaced but iridodonesis occurring

Another complication in the presentation of a dog with lens luxation is that the condition does appear in breeds other that the terriers in which it is a clearly inherited trait. And even more confusingly, while glaucoma can,

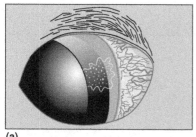

(a)

Signs of subluxation:

- Aphakic crescent
- Possible vitreal tag in anterior chamber

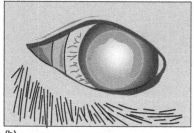

(b)

Signs of primary luxation

- Lens obvious in anterior chamber
- Pupil block glaucoma
- Breeds–terrier and border collie

Note: reflected light often outlines the lens in the anterior chamber

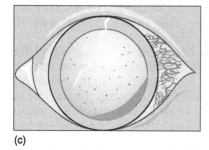

(c)

Signs of secondary luxation

- Glaucoma with enlarged globe
- Descemet's fracture
- Breeds predisposed to glaucoma

Figure 8.1 Subluxation of lens

and often does, occur secondary to lens luxation, lens luxation itself can occur secondary to glaucoma. Thus the management of a luxated lens is not always lentectomy. When the luxation occurs as a result of globe enlargement removal of the lens will do nothing to ameliorate ocular signs. The glaucoma which has caused buphthalmos must originate elsewhere. This may be at the iridocorneal angle, a primary goniodysgenesis glaucoma or perhaps through peripheral anterior synechiae following uveitis. The differentiation of whether glaucoma follows lens luxation, or lens luxation follows glaucoma, relies on two questions.

- Is there a reason for glaucoma other than the lens luxation?

- What is the primary ocular defect – zonular breakdown or globe enlargement following glaucoma?

This calls, as do all ophthalmological questions, for a close examination of the globe. Look in particular for

- the position of the lens – use a slit beam if possible
- a possible area of corneal oedema in the central cornea suggestive of current or previous anterior lens luxation
- vitreal strands protruding into the aqueous
- any signs of subluxation in the other eye
- the size of the globe – visual inspection and the presence of Haab's striae or Descemet's fractures. These are caused by

the posterior influx of aqueous humour into the stroma at the sites of rupture in Descemet's membrane. An enlarged globe with an acute lens luxation suggests that the lens luxation is secondary

- any other signs of disease producing glaucoma – inflammation or neoplasia.

In the cat, lens luxation is almost always seen following glaucoma, uveitis or rarely trauma (Olivero et al 1991). The mechanism of zonule breakdown subsequent to uveitis is unclear but this link with other ocular abnormalities shows, yet again, the importance of assessing the whole eye and not just focusing on the obvious abnormality. The link with uveitis is noteworthy, both because it shows the importance of assessing the underlying cause of intra-ocular inflammation in such cases (see Chapter 6) and also because the anterior segment in such cases is already in a state of inflammatory activity. Entry into the globe in such circumstances should not be attempted without considerable local (topical) and systemic anti-inflammatory medication before surgery.

8.2 Diabetic cataract®

As noted above, it might seem surprising to class any cataract as an emergency, but from time to time owners fail to recognise early signs of lenticular opacification in their animal and see a complete cataract as a sudden change. The animal's visual disturbance is the first sign they notice and the white cataract the second. With such unobservant owners the cataract may be the first sign they notice of their animal's diabetes, polyuria and polydipsia having been missed or ignored. Cataract can occur very rapidly in an uncontrolled diabetic animal. The markedly increased glucose levels in the lens swamp the classic Ebden Myerhoff metabolic pathway. This allows excess glucose to be metabolized by the enzyme aldose reductase which is normally not able to act on the sugar at low concentrations, given its lower affinity for the substrate. Aldose reductase converts glucose into sorbitol and this insoluble sugar creates an osmotic gradient across the cell membrane and leads to lens fibre swelling, and then

irreversible opacification. Management of this situation is lentectomy by extracapsular extraction, or more frequently today phaco-emulsification. The important factor here is recognition that the cataract is secondary to diabetes: every cataract case should undergo a full haematological and serum biochemistry profile as a key part of the work up before surgical treatment.

8.3 Lens capsule rupture and phacoanaphylactic uveitis®

In circumstances where lenticular trauma liberates lens proteins, severe, almost anaphylactic changes in the eye are seen, termed phacoanaphylactic or phacoclastic uveitis. In the majority of these instances rupture of the lens capsule by a penetrating foreign body is responsible for release of lens material. A typical setting is a thorn or cat-claw injury to the globe, typically through the cornea. Thus in any case of corneal damage it is important to assess the anterior surface of the lens capsule. If a means of magnification is not to hand, fluorescence such as a Wood's lamp in a dark room will help detect any damage: the lens will autofluoresce to some degree, aiding observation of capsular rupture or perforation.

In one interesting situation trauma from within the lens itself causes capsular rupture. This is the case of lens-induced uveitis in the rabbit where the protozoan parasite *Encephalitozoon cuniculi*, transmitted vertically from mother to offspring in utero, is found in the lens of the young adult rabbit. In some circumstances these protozoan larvae rupture the capsule and a lens-induced uveitis follows. This does not appear to be a phacoanaphylactic uveitis as such, rather a phacoclastic inflammation with a white inflammatory focus occurring in the anterior chamber. This must be differentiated from a *Pasteurella multocida* uveitis which could give a similar white purulent inflammatory deposit. Discussion of such cases is beyond the remit of this volume, since these animals are not generally presented as emergencies but rather as chronic problems.

In cases of lens rupture aggressive anti-inflammatory treatment is advised, such as topical dexamethasone or prednisolone acetate 3–4 times daily. Removal of the lens at this stage by phaco-emulsification is probably the best treatment option while medical treatment with anti-inflammatories may be sufficient in mild cases. In many cases a severe uveitis with secondary glaucoma supervenes and the removal of the lens by phaco-emulsification is probably the therapeutic route to be recommended.

Chapter 9

Retina and vitreous

9.1 Retinal detachment

Retinal detachment presents as an emergency when it occurs bilaterally with sudden visual impairment and often complete blindness. Several systemic or ocular conditions may be the cause of a retinal detachment. A key aim

Emergency management of retinal detachment

1. Perform full ophthalmic examination
2. Define whether detachment is rhegmatogenous (with retinal tear) or non-rhegmatogenous
3. Determine whether systemic disease (hypertension, inflammatory focus etc.) is present
4. Manage hypertension with amlodipine per os
5. Manage posterior uveitis with prednisolone per os

Prognostic indicators in retinal detachment

1. Prolonged detachment before diagnosis a poor prognostic sign, as retinal atrophy often occurs with time
2. Rhegmatogenous detachment more difficult to treat than non-rhegmatogenous
3. Association with hypertension a good prognostic sign, as medical treatment often resolves detachment in such cases
4. Association with posterior uveitis a poorer sign, as complete resolution is less common

of full diagnostic work up in retinal detachment is thus the investigation of whether and which of these diseases is the cause of the detachment. On the other hand, there are retinal detachments which are the result of intra-ocular abnormalities such as anomalies of the vitreous, retina, optic disc or choroid. For this reason a full ocular examination is mandatory, this including scleral indentation, in order to visualize the peripheral retina where many tears leading to detachment occur. Sometimes it may be difficult to see what is actually happening in the eye, as extensive haemorrhages after the detachment may impair visual diagnosis. Ocular ultrasound equipment provides very valuable information in such circumstances. The typical features of a retinal detachment are shown in Figure 9.1 and Table 9.1.

One systemic disease which may be an underlying cause is hypertension, either alone or associated with chronic renal failure or hyperthyroidism, more so in the cat than the dog. An ocular condition leading to detachment which may be part of a systemic disease is posterior uveitis. While this can occur on its own, it can be part of a systemic auto-immune condition such as uveodermatological syndrome (VKH or Vogt-Koyanagi-Harada-like disease) in which peri-ocular loss of pigmentation (poliosis and vitiligo) is seen. Retinal detachment can occur as part of a recognized ocular syndrome in a specific breed such as retinal dysplasia in the Bedlington or Sealyham terrier, or Collie eye

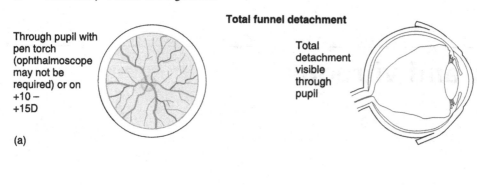

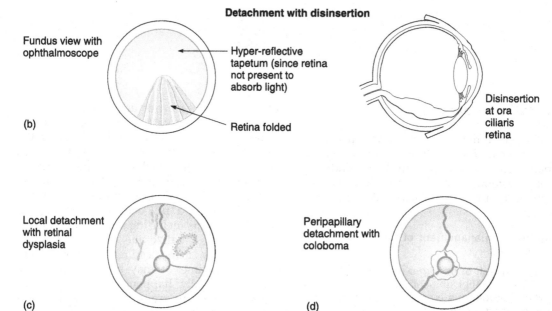

Figure 9.1 (a) Total funnel detachment visible through pupil; (b) detachment with disinsertion; (c) partial detachment with retinal dysplasia; (d) partial detachment with optic nerve coloboma

Table 9.1 Differential diagnosis of retinal detachment

Pathogenesis of detachment

Exudative detachment	– inflammatory or exudative fluid between neuroretina and RPE
Rhegmatogenous detachment	– retinal tear causes detachment
Traction detachment	– vitreal bands pull neuroretina away

Differential diagnosis

Exudative detachment:	– Uveitis Hypertension
Rhegmatogenous detachment	– Trauma Detachment associated with hypermature cataract
Traction detachment	– Trauma Post-inflammatory

anomaly in the Collie breeds. It can occur following a space-occupying lesion such as a tumour in the retrobulbar space or can follow trauma. With regard to the globe itself detachments can occur at the rim of a coloboma of the optic disc, these being related to anatomical abnormalities of retinal adhesion at the edge of the optic disc.

The relationship between the vitreous and the retina are important in maintaining the retina correctly positioned. Vitreal degeneration, which occurs in many older animals, can lead to vitreal cavitation with liquefaction (synchysis scintillans). This condition should be differentiated from asteroid hyalosis and posterior vitreal detachment. Here the attachment of the vitreous to the inner retina fails. In the majority of animals this goes unnoticed and causes no visual disturbance. It may, however, cause peripheral retinal tears, which can extend centrally to give significant visual disturbance. Rhegmatogenous retinal detachments, i.e. those associated with retinal tears, most often occur between the neuroretina and the retinal pigment epithelium as the connection between these two structures is tenuous. Non-rhegmatogenous detachments occurring after serous exudation into this intraretinal space (commonly but rather confusingly termed the subretinal space) also manifest at this weak point of the retina. Cataracts and lens luxations may cause retinal tears; retinal detachment may be a complication of cataract surgery in animals.

Some detachments associated with a systemic problem such as hypertension occur almost simultaneously in both eyes. Alternatively it may be that one detachment has preceded the other by some considerable period, and that the visual deficit is not noticed until the second eye is affected and the animal becomes completely blind. By that stage treatment is difficult and often not particularly effective for the eye with the long-standing detachment, but certainly still worth attempting for that eye and also for the eye with the recent detachment.

Ideally, blood pressure measurement should be undertaken using either an oscillometric sphygomomanometer or a doppler unit which, being relatively cheap, should be available in every larger practice for monitoring blood pressure during anaesthesia as well as the less for diagnosis of hypertensive retinopathy. Hypertensive cats are often in early to moderate or severe renal failure or may be typical of feline hyperthyroidism, with signs such as weight loss and tachycardia. Amlodipine in the cat (0.625 mg daily) often results in retinal re-attachment and restored vision, but management of the underlying cause is vital.

Other causes of retinal detachments presenting as emergencies can be rapid fluid overload in renally compromised animals in which case bullous retinal detachments can be seen (Martin 1999).

9.1.1 Examination of the animal with a retinal detachment

The fundus is readily examined by ophthalmoscopy using either direct or indirect methods. With direct fundoscopy the retina can be seen in focus only with the direct ophthalmoscope on a setting of over 0 D, indicating that the retina is placed anterior to its normal position at the most posterior aspect of the globe. With binocular indirect ophthalmoscopy a three-dimensional view of the retina is obtained showing clearly that it is detached. When the retina balloons to the front of the vitreous is readily visible even without an ophthamoscope, through the widely dilated pupils resulting from lack of visual stimulus. It usually looks like a very fine silk veil floating behind the lens. As noted above scleral indentation allows a complete view of the peripheral retina. Local anaesthetic should be applied to the eye and a scleral indentor used gently to push the globe inwards behind the limbus. Using the head-mounted binocular indirect ophthalmoscope and full mydriasis, the portion of the peripheral retina indented can be visualized and checked for retinal degeneration or retinal tears.

The eye with a retinal detachment developing as a consequence of hypertension may often have several tell-tale signs before complete detachment occurs. Retinal vessels may be tortuous and appear like a chain of sausages with lengths of vessel constriction and dilation. Retinal haemorrhages and/or vascular exudates may be seen with small areas of flat detachment occurring before bullous exudative detachments lead on to complete detachment.

When unilateral detachment is seen, useful diagnostic information can be gained from examination of the fellow eye. Often this has disease at an earlier stage, in a progressive disease such as hypertension. Alternatively it may be that the other eye shows signs of a condition with multiple ocular features one of which can lead to retinal detachment, such as occurs in retinal dysplasia or Collie eye anomaly. In the former the apparently unaffected eye may have retinal folds or multifocal areas of dysplasia; in the latter there may be a coloboma or chorioretinal dysplasia.

In animals, particularly cats, in which a hypertensive aetiology is likely, indirect blood pressure measurement is essential for a full diagnostic work up. Doppler sphygmomanometry has been reported in dogs and cats as being successful, although the more reliable (and more costly) method of oscillometric measurement reported recently gives more reproducible results (Bodey and Michell 1996). Certainly direct measurement requiring an arterial line is not necessary to measure blood pressure in cats and dogs now, and measurement of mean blood pressure should be within the grasp of any interested veterinarian. Time is required to ensure that several reproducible results from a calm animal are obtained. The normal measurements reported in the literature can be found in Bodey et al. 1994, Bodey and Michell 1996. The differences in normal values between different breeds of dog should be noted. A consistently high reading in a dog or cat should alert one to the likelihood of a hypertensive detachment, although such a finding in an animal with a detachment does not necessarily prove a causative relationship. Essential hypertension, although common in people, is not seen frequently in dogs and cats. Animals with a finding of hypertension should be investigated for renal disease and, in the case of cats, also for hyperthyroidism.

9.1.2 Treatment of retinal detachment secondary to hypertension

In the absence of renal disease or hyperthyroidism, hypertension may be treated with a calcium channel blocker such as amlodipine (Istin). For cats 0.625 mg s.i.d. (⅛ of a 5 mg tablet of amlodipine) in the evening is sufficient to give a significant reduction in blood pressure (Henik et al. 1997). It is sometimes impractical to prescribe ⅛ of a tablet and 1.25 mg (¼ tablet) has yielded no side effects in our experience. The frequency of spontaneous retinal re-attachment after normalization of blood pressure is difficult to assess, but is high enough to convince that the treatment is worth pursuing. In many cases while one retina is chronically detached, the second eye has a recent detachment giving rise to the total blindness which alerts the owner and leads to presentation of the animal.

The authors have seen amlopidine therapy used to good effect in cats with hypertensive retinopathy and renal disease. Lowering the blood pressure will have beneficial effects on the chronic renal failure as well. The chronically detached retina may not be functional even if re-attachment occurs, but the acutely detached retina often regains useful function after antihypertensive treatment has been successfully implemented.

9.1.3 Treatment of retinal detachment in posterior uveitis

Retinal detachment in a case such as a Vogt-Koyanagi-Harada-like syndrome in the dog is related to inflammatory changes causing effusion into the subretinal space. The breeds found to be affected with VKH-syndrome include Akika, Siberian husky, Chow chow, Golden retriever, Samoyed, Irish setter, Shetland sheepdog, Saint Bernard, Old English sheepdog and Australian shepherd (Martin 1999). The main presenting signs include sudden blindness, bullous retinal detachments and secondary glaucoma. In such cases aggressive anti-inflammatory treatment with systemic prednisolone at 1.5 mg/kg or with azathioprine at 2 mg/kg s.i.d. reducing to 0.5 mg/kg. Forty-eight hours is required for steroid effects although azathioprine requires a longer period to gain efficacy.

Fungal disease can be a cause of retinal detachment following granulomatous retinitis or choroiditis associated with systemic infection with organisms such as *Crypotococcus neoformans* or *Neosporum canis*. Diagnosis can be by visualization of organisms on a vitreous tap or by serum antigen detection. Treatment is with agents such as itraconazole (Carlton et al. 1976, Jacobs et al. 1997).

9.1.4 Treatment of idiopathic retinal detachment

Retinal detachment which has occurred without an obvious predisposing cause may be rhegmatogenous or non-rhegmatogenous, see section 1.9.1. The treatment of these two forms differs in some important respects.

Rhegmatogenous detachments are best treated surgically with one of three techniques. Scleral contour can be altered to bring the sclera in apposition to the detached retina by scleral buckling. Alternatively re-attachment can be achieved by production of a chorioretinal scar though cryosurgery, diathermy or transpupillary photocoagulation. Thirdly subretinal fluid can be drained trans-sclerally. Recently complex vitreoretinal surgerical techniques used in human ophthalmology have been performed in the dog. All of these techniques clearly should be attempted only at a specialist referral clinic. The reader is thus directed to more comprehensive texts and papers in the specialist literature for information regarding specialist vitreoretinal surgery (Smith 1999, Vainisi and Packo 1995).

9.2 Sudden acquired retinal degeneration

The diagnosis of sudden acquired retinal degeneration (SARD) is based on a history of sudden unexplained visual deterioration and a complete absence of retinal response on electroretinography. Performing an electroretinogram (ERG) in such cases might seem academic as there is no treatment for SARD. The test is, however, essential to differentiate from problems where the ERG does show retinal activity and a central cause for the blindness must be sought.

While the history of sudden visual loss might seem a clear one, investigation of a number of cases in our clinics and the findings of several others show that what is termed sudden visual loss can cover quite a range of circumstances. Some animals are visual one minute and then blind a moment or two afterwards, this state remaining permanently. This severe manifestation remains however quite rare. The majority of dogs finally diagnosed as having SARD have suffered a rapidly progressing but not ultra-rapid deterioration in sight, perhaps over a matter of a few days. It is the ERG which determines the diagnosis in these cases.

No mechanism is understood for this sudden visual deprivation and no identical condition is seen in man, or apparently in animals, other than the dog. A similar condition in man known as cancer-associated retinopathy occurs, particularly with small cell carcinoma of the lung. These patients can suffer with sudden loss of vision and there is an associated finding of circulating antibodies to recoverin, a molecule in the visual pathway which has antigenic similarities to a molecule found in small cell carcinoma cells. No association with a neoplastic process has been reported in dogs with SARD, but many have hypothalamopituitary axis defects such as Cushing's syndrome or at least abnormal ACTH stimulation tests (Van der Woerdt et al. 1991, Mattson et al. 1992). Dogs presenting with SARD should thus be evaluated for such endocrine abnormalities.

Chapter 10

Optic nerve

10.1 Optic neuritis®

Optic neuritis generally presents as sudden blindness and as such the differential diagnosis includes sudden acquired retinal degeneration and central blindness. Here the clinical feature allowing a diagnosis to be made is optic nerve swelling. The problem is that the appearance of optic nerve head swelling is very difficult, if not impossible, to differentiate from the papilloedema which can be seen with a space-occupying lesion that could present as central blindness.

Emergency management of optic neuritis

1. Perform full ophthalmic examination
2. Specifically evaluate pupillary light reflexes and swinging light test
3. Evaluate other neurological parameters with suspicion of diseases such as GME
4. Give systemic steroid at 1–2 mg/kg

Prognostic indicators in optic neuritis

1. Duration of blindness an important prognostic sign, more than five days poor
2. Degree of optic nerve swelling and haemorrhage potentially a poor sign although can resolve on aggressive treatment
3. Degree of optic disc pallor an important sign as this suggests the onset of optic atrophy

Generally, however, the difference is that optic neuritis produces visual dysfunction, whereas papilloedema does not unless resulting from an intracranial lesion which concurrently causes blindness. Optic nerve head swelling is characterized by a domed enlargement of the optic papilla with a fuzzy indistinct border to the disc and surface haemorrhages. It is the authors' experience that optic neuritis is more likely to present with haemorrhage at the optic disc than is papilloedema, although vessels of the optic disc are engorged in both. To date, however, we have no definitive evidence that this is the case.

The big question centres around what other neurological inflammatory foci may be present. A full neurological examination is mandatory and the use of computerized tomography (CT) or magnetic resonance imaging (MRI) is invaluable to show if other inflammatory lesions are occurring intracranially. Optic neuritis occurs in humans as part of multiple sclerosis and in dogs as a manifestation of granulomatous meningo-encephalitis (GME). It is thus essential that other manifestations of GME be investigated. Whether other neurological lesions are found or not, the treatment is systemic steroid at an anti-inflammatory dose and this may need to continue for a significant time if recurrence of blindness on cessation of treatment is to be avoided. If the patient cannot be seen by a veterinary ophthalmologist for electroretinography, or referral for

CT/MRI, the veterinary surgeon has the vision of the animal to gain and nothing to lose by using anti inflammatory agents.

Retrobulbar optic neuritis has the same effects on vision without the fundus changes seen where the optic nerve head is involved; high resolution retrobulbar ultrasound can be useful in defining it. The incidence of this condition is not clear, but apparently low.

10.2 Central blindness®

Blindness not associated with disease of the globe or the extracranial optic nerve can be associated with intracranial mass lesions. These may have effects on vision predominantly through two mechanisms. One is a rise in intracranial pressure while the other is direct effect on the visual pathways. The most common lesion producing an acute decrease in vision is a tumour at the level of the optic chiasm causing chiasmal compression. Most often these are pituitary macro-adenomas which may, or may not be associated with hormonal imbalances and such obvious changes as polydipsia and polyuria. All these intracranial lesions require a neurological as well as an ophthalmological, and quite possibly also an oncological referral.

Conclusions

Emergency ophthalmology is an exciting discipline in which, while life is rarely at stake, recovery of a painfree visual eye is often in the hands of the veterinary surgeon first seeing the case: an intensely miotic pupil is best dealt with at the first consultation; a correct first apposition of lid edges in a traumatic lid lesion is critical; a delay in treatment of an acute glaucoma will almost inevitably lead to permanent blindness. Thus it is not only the specialist who should be well equipped for dealing with the ocular emergency but also veterinarians in first-opinion practice.

There is a balance to be struck between the step-by-step approach to dealing with these problems, as shown through the flow diagrams here, and the more detailed background knowledge contained in the text. The latter helps cement an understanding of the pathogenic mechanisms occurring in disease conditions and thus the ameliorative effects of optimal treatment regimens. It is hoped that combining these approaches will aid the reader in dealing with the wide range of ocular emergencies seen in veterinary practice.

David Williams 2002

Diagnostic methods used in veterinary ophthalmology

1. Performing the Schirmer tear test

The pack is opened and the little snip is bent inside the plastic pack. With one hand the lower eyelid is everted and the snip is placed like a hook over the eyelid margin. The eyelid is returned to rest on the eye. Care must be taken to avoid the test strip falling out once placed, and if the animal is agitated the eyelids may be held slightly closed to prevent loss of the strip.

After one minute the STT-strip is removed and the reading noted. The STT-strip may have a colour indicator (Schering-Plough/Eagle Vision). If no markings are on the STT-strip the length of wetted paper must be measured against the STT-strip pack or a ruler.

With a little practice the clinician will be able to place two strips in each eye at the same time and thus perform the Schirmer tear test in both eyes simultaneously.

While a number of reports have documented different ranges of normal values in various species, it can be said that a Schirmer tear test over 15 mm/min demonstrates a normal tear production in the cat or dog In the dog a value under 5 mm/min is indicative of keratoconjunctivitis sicca and a value between 5 and 10 mm/min suggests early or mild changes in the aqueous component of tears. In the cat some animals with a healthy ocular surface have very low readings but in general the same figures can

be applied. Small mammals have, understandably, lower tear production and in some species such as the rabbit the little research carried out demonstrates substantial difference in STT values between different breeds.

2. Measurement of the intra-ocular pressure (IOP) with Schiotz tonometer

While the optimal tonometer for small animal use is considered to be the Tonopen applanation tonometer, the much cheaper Schiotz indentation tonometer can, with practice, be used accurately to assess intra-ocular pressure.

An anaesthetic is instilled topically onto the cornea. The nose of the animal is held in an upright position so the cornea is horizontal. Then the Schiotz tonometer is applied to the cornea and the reading is noted. It is important that the foot of the tonometer is on the central cornea as the identation of the sclera will cause a faulty reading of the intra-ocular pressure.

The Schiotz tonometer is an indentation tonometer, where hardness of the eye is inversely proportional to the indentation (i.e. a higher reading indicates a lower intra-ocular pressure and a low reading indicates high intra-ocular pressure). The reading on the scale is correlated to the intra-ocular pressure by using a table. Friedenwald's research in the 1950s resulted in a table for human values. (Friedenwald 1957). Since then papers have been published proposing the use of different tables for Schiotz tonometry on the canine eye (Peiffer et al. 1977a, Peiffer et al. 1977b), but the latest conclusions are that the original Friedenwald table revised in 1955 (Friedenwald 1957) is the most accurate and applicable to the dog (Miller and Pickett 1992a). The Friedenwald Table from 1955 is shown below for weights 5.5 g, 7.5 g and 10.0 g, and may also be used in the cat (Miller and Pickett 1992b), although Schiotz tonometry is more easily performed in the dog.

The optimal method of using the Schiotz tonometer takes several measurements with different weights which make possible a more accurate estimation of the intra-ocular pressure. Separate readings with the 5.5 g, 7.5 g and 10 g weights can be used with the graph depicted below using data from the original Friedenwald table. The best estimate of intra ocular pressure is the y axis intercept.

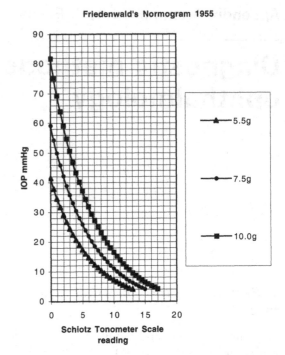

Friedenwald's Normogram 1955

Ocular dictionary

Acuity: *the ability to see the details of an object separately and unblurred*

Aphakic: *without lens – as in aphakic crescent in lens luxation*

Asteroid hyalosis: *deposition of chlolesterol/calcium deposits in vitreous humour. See Synchysis scillitans*

Blepharospasm: *excessive blinking, tonic or clonic spasm of the m. orbicularis oculi. Associated with irritation or pain of the eye, most often corneal pain*

Buphthalmos: *enlargement of the globe due to chronic glaucoma*

CAI (carbonic anhydrase inhibitor): *drug that reduces aqueous humour formation in the treatment of glaucoma*

Cataract: *an opacity within the lens. Must be differentiated from nuclear sclerosis (q.v.)*

Chalazion: *chronic inflammatory granuloma resulting from retention of secretion from a meibomian gland*

Chemosis: *oedema of the conjunctiva*

Chronic superficial keratitis (pannus): *superficial predominantly lymphocytic inflammation of the cornea seen as a distinct entity in dog breeds such as the German Shepherd and Collie*

Ciliary flush: *a diffuse, rose-red coloration surrounding the cornea as a result of congestion of the branches of the anterior ciliary arteries, in cyclitis, iridocyclitis or deep keratitis*

Cornea: *the transparent front part of the eye joining the sclera at the limbus*

Descemetocoele: *a forward building of Descemet's membrane through a weakened or absent corneal stroma as a result of trauma or a deep corneal ulcer*

Distichiasis: *hairs growing from the meibomian glands*

Ectopic cilia: *hairs growing from areas that should be devoid of hair. Usually on the palpebral conjunctiva, and with origins in the meibomian glands as these evolutionarily were hair follicles*

Ectropion: *eversion of the eyelid margin. Most often seen in giantdog breeds such as Saint Bernard, Chow Chow etc. Often the patients have a chronic exposure conjunctivitis*

Enophthalmos: *recession of the eyeball into the orbit*

Entropion: *turning inward (inversion) of the eyelid. Most commonly the lower eyelid, and often associated with trichiasis*

Enucleation: *surgical removal of the globe*

ERG (electroretinography): *an electrophysiological method of measuring the retinal response to light*

Evisceration: *surgical removal of the contents of the globe followed in most cases by implantation of a silicone sphere as a prosthesis*

Exenteration: *surgical removal of the globe and extra-ocular structures. Indication for extenteration is infection of the eye and orbital tissues and/or metastatic neoplasia*

Exophthalmos: *an abnormal protrusion of the eyeball from the orbit. Physiological in brachycephalic breeds*

Facet: *depression in the cornea covered by corneal epithelium and seen after corneal ulceration with loss of corneal stromal tissue*

Flare (aqueous flare, Tyndall's effect): *the scattering of a thin beam of light as it transverses the anterior chamber, caused by an increase in the* protein content of the aqueous humour. A sign of uveitis. May be graded 1 to 4

Follicular conjunctivitis (plasmoma): *conjunctivitis often seen in conjunction with pannus, in which lymphoid follicles give a nodular appearance*

Fornix (of the conjunctiva): *the part of the conjunctiva that joins the palpebral and the bulbar conjunctiva, and which is unattached to the eyelid or the eyeball. Much deeper in the dog than in the human, it may be difficult to obtain cells from the fornix for exfoliative cytology*

Glaucoma: *increased intra-ocular pressure. Often manifests with dilated pupil, negative PLR, corneal oedema and potentially breaks in descemets membranes (Haab's striae)*

Gonioscopy: *optical examination of the irido-corneal angle using a goniolens and a means of magnification*

Haab's striae: *Breaks in descemets membrane causing aqueous humour to impede into the corneal stroma.The breaks are caused by globe stretching. See Glaucoma*

Hordeolum: *external hordeolum is a purulent infection of a sebaceous gland along the eyelid margin. Internal is an acute purulent infection of a meibomian gland*

Horner's syndrome: *sympathetic denervation to the eye resulting in miosis, ptosis and enophthalmos*

Hyphaema: *accumulation of red blood cells/blood in the anterior chamber. Usually associated with coagulopathy, uveitis, feline hypertension or ocular trauma*

Hypopyon: *accumulation of pus in the anterior chamber. The pus usually sinks to the bottom filling the lower angle of the anterior chamber*

Iridodonesis: *trembling of the iris when the eye is moved (by examiner). Associated with lens luxation*

Keratic precipitates (KPs): *cellular deposits on the posterior surface of the cornea, usually in association with iritis or iridocyclitis*

Keratoconjunctivitis sicca (KCS): *decreased quantitative tear production resulting in pathological changes of the cornea and conjunctiva*

Lagophthalmos: *the eyelids do not meet when supposed to be closed. Test by applying touch to lateral canthus. If lagophthalmos is present the central cornea may be exposed during sleep, thus dehydrating. Often a central corneal ulcer is concurrent with lagophthalmos*

Lens-induced uveitis (LIU): *uveitis induced by leakage of lens protein*

Limbus: *the junction of the cornea and sclera*

Lymphocytic/plasmacytic conjunctivitis: *conjunctivitis often seen with pannus in which lymphoid follicles give a nodular appearance or, in less severe cases, a generalized red conjunctiva*

Meibomianitis: *inflammation of the meibomian glands resulting in qualitative tear film disease and increased evaporation of tears*

Miosis: *decrease in pupil size. Seen in uveitis and in Horner's syndrome (q.v.)*

Mydriasis: *increase in pupil size. Often seen in glaucoma or in nervous animals, particularly cats*

Nuclear sclerosis: *the natural ageing of the lens causes impaction/hardening of the nucleus of the lens, as the growth of lens fibres continues throughout life*

Pannus: *see Chronic superficial keratitis*

Paracentesis: *sampling aqueous humour from the anterior chamber by means of a hypodermic needle inserted at the limbus*

Photophobic: *an abnormal intolerance or fear of light. Often associated with uveitis*

Plasmoma: *see Follicular conjunctivitis*

PRA (progressive retinal atrophy): *a congenital progressive blindness found in a number of canine breeds and the Abyssinian cat. Diagnosis is by ERG (q.v.). Ophthalmoscopically retinal vessels are attenuated and the retina is hyper-reflective*

Proptosis: *protrusion of the globe beyond the eyelids (see Exophthalmos)*

Ptosis: *drooping of the eyelid. Usually a sign of neurological deficit as seen in Horner's syndrome or facial nerve paralysis. May also be seen in enophthalmos*

SARD (sudden acquired retinal degeneration): *blindness characterized by rapid onset and flat electroretinogram – of unknown cause*

Staphyloma: *a bulging or protrusion of the cornea or the sclera usually containing adherent uveal tissue*

Synchysis scillitans: *liquefaction of the vitreous, to be differentiated from asteroid hyalosis. If the head of the animal is shaken synchysis scillitans will show an appearance of bright dots falling from the sky. In asteroid hyalosis the white opacities are fixed within the corpus vitreous and only vibrate after a shaking*

Synnechae: *anterior, posterior. Adhesion of the iris to the cornea or to the capsule of the crystalline lens*

Tarsorraphy: *tying the eyelid margins together with sutures, mostly applying horizontal mattress sutures or a horizontal Lembert suture pattern*

Trichiasis: *inversion of eyelashes thus touching the eyeball and causing irritaion, most often associated with normal hair in an abnormal position, such as in entropion*

Uvea: *iris, ciliary body and choroid. Anterior uvea: iris and ciliary body. Posterior uvea: choroid*

VKH (Vogt-Koyonagi-Harada syndrome): *an inherited auto-immune disease, where melanin is thought to be the antigen. It is phagocytosed, resulting in posterior uveitis, poliuosis and vitiligo with depigmentation of peri-ocular and other structures*

International ocular drug formulary

Trade	Generic	Formulation	Company	Action
Acular	Ketorolac	0.5% drops	Allergan	NSAID
AK-CON™	Naphazoline HCl	0.1% drops	Akorn	Anti-H
AK-NaCl®	Sodium Chloride	5% ointment	Akorn	Osmotic
AK-TAINE®	Proparacaine HCl	0.5%	Akorn	Anaesthetic
AK-TROL	Dexamethasone 0.1%, Neomycin sulphate, Polymixin B		Akorn	Steroid A-pos/neg
Albalon 0.1%	Naphazoline HCl	0.1% drops	Allergan	Anti-H
Alcaine	Proparacaine HCl	0.5% drops	Alcon	Anaesthetic
Alomide	Lodoxamide	0.1% drops	Alcon	Anti-H
Amethocaine	Amethocaine	0.5% drops	generic	Anaesthetic
Atropine	Atropine	0.5–1% drops	generic	Antimuscarinic
Aureomycin	Chlortetracycline	1% ointment	Lederle	A-pos/neg Chla
Azopt	Brinzolamide	1% drops	Alcon	CAI
Bacitracin	Bacitracin	500–1000 units/ml	Upjohn	A-pos (Staph)
Betnesol	Betamethasone	0.1% drops	Medeva	Steroid
Betnesol-N	Betamethasone and neomycin		Medeva	Steroid + A
Cepravin	Cephalonium	8% ointment	Schering-Plough Animal Health	A-pos/neg
Chloromycetin	Chloramphenicol	1% ointment	Goldshield	A-pos/neg
Ciloxan	Ciprofloxacin	0.3% drops	Alcon	A-pos/neg
Ciproxin	Ciprofloxacin	2 mg/ml 50 ml bottle	Bayfarm	A-pos/neg
Daranide	Dichlorphenamide	50 mg tabs	Merck & Co	CAI
Diamox	Acetazolamide	125/250/500 mg tabs	Wyeth Lederle	CAI
Exocin	Ofloxacin	0.3% drops	Allergan	A-pos/neg
Finadyne	Flunixine meglumine	Inject/granules	Schering-Plough Animal Health	NSAID
Fluorescein	Fluorescein	1 or 2% minim drops	Chauvin	Dye
FML	Fluorometholone	0.1% drops	Allergan	Steroid
Fucithalmic Vet	Fusidic acid	1% ointment	LEO	A-pos (Staph)
Garamycin	Gentamicin	3%	Schering	A-neg
Genticin	Gentamicin	0.3%	Roche	A-neg
Glauctabs	Methazolamide	tabs	Akorn	CAI
Glaupax	Acetazolamide	125/250 mg tabs	Orion Pharma	CAI
Herplex	Idoxuridine	0.1% drops	Allergan	V-H
Humorsol	Demecarium bromide	0.25% drops	Merck & Co	Parasympatho-mimetics
Intron-A	Interferon alpha-2b	5x10E6 IU/ml	Schering-Plough	V-H

Trade	Generic	Formulation	Company	Action
Istin	Amlodipine	5 mg, 10 mg tab	Pfizer	Ca-channel blocker
Ketofen	Ketoprofen	5 mg tabs, inj	Fort Dodge Animal Health	NSAID
Lacri-lube	White petrolatum, mineral oil, lanolin derivatives		Allergan	Artificial tears/ocular lubricant
Lissamine green	Lissamine green	Dry powder	Sigma-Aldrich	Dye
Livosten	Levocabastine	0.05% drops	Ciba-vision	Antihistamine
Lysine	L-lysine	250 mg tabs	generic	V-H
Mannitol	Mannitol	Fluid for i.v.	generic	Osmotic
Maxidex	Dexamethasone	Drops	Alcon	Steroid
Maxitrol	Dexamethasone 0.1%, Neomycin Sulphate, Polymixin B Sulphate	Drops	Alcon	Steroid A-pos/neg
Methazol-amide USP	Methazolamide	25 mg and 50 mg	Lederle	CAI
Muro-128	Sodium chloride	5% ointment	Bauch & Lomb	Osmotic
Mydriacyl	Tropicamide	0.5%	Alcon	Antimuscarinic
Nebcin (a)	Tobramycin	40 mg/ml inj	Lilly	A-neg
Neptazane	Methazolamide	Tabs	Stortz Ophthalmics	CAI
Norvasc	Amlodipine	2.5 mg, 5 mg, 10 mg tabs	Pfizer	Ca-channel blocker
Ocufen	Flubiprofen	0.03% drops	Allergan	NSAID
Ophthaine	Proparacaine HCl	0.5% drops	Bristol-Myers	Anaesthetic
Optimmune	Cyclosporine	0.2% ointment	Schering-Plough	T-cell inhib
Oralcon	Dichlorphenamide	50 mg tab	Alcon	CAI
Phenylephrine	Phenylephrine	10% drops	generic	Sympathomimetic
Pilocarpine	Pilocarpine	0.5-3% drops	generic	Miotic
Pred forte	Prednisolone acetate	1% drops	Allergan	Steroid
Rimadyl	Carprofen	Tab/inj	Pfizer	NSAID
Rose Bengal	Rose Bengal	1% minim vials	Chauvin	Dye
Sandimune	Cyclosporine	50 mg/ml 1 ml/5 ml amps	Novartis	T-cell inhibitor
Stroxil	Idoxuridine	0.1% drops	Smith Kline & French	V-H
Tobrex	Tobramycin	0.3% drops	Alcon	A-neg
Trusopt	Dorzolamide	2% drops	MSD	CAI
Vira A	Vidarabine	3% ointment	Parke Davis	V-H
Viroptic	Trifluridine	1% drops	Borroughs Wellcome	V-H
Vistamethasone	Betamethasone	0.1% drops	Martindale	Steroid
Voltarol/Voltaren	Diclofenac	0.1% drops	Ciba-Vision	NSAID
Xalatan	Latanoprost	50 µg/ml	Pharmacia & Upjohn	Prostaglandin analogue
Zinacef	Cefuroxime	250/750 mg amp	Glaxo Wellcome	A-pos
Zovirax	Acyclovir	3% eye ointment 200 mg, 400 mg and 800 mg tabs	Glaxo-Wellcome	V-H

Abbreviations
NSAID: Non steroid anti-inflammatory drug
Amp: ampoules
A: antibiotic
A-neg: antibiotic for Gram-negative infection
A-pos: antibiotic for Gram-positive infection
A-pos/neg: antibiotic for Gram-negative and Gram-positive infection
CAI: carbonic anhydrase inhibitor
Chla: Chlamydia
Dye: ocular diagnostic dye
Staph: staphylococcus
V-H: antiviremica against herpes-virus (including stimulation of immune response)

Varieties of the same drug sold under different names are included in the above table. Most of these (generic) drugs are from Akorn, as this is the largest generic eye drug company in the US. In other parts of the world most of the products may be made up in local pharmacies or hospital pharmacies if the original product is not used.

General instructions for eye medication
Only apply one drop to each eye. Always wait a minimum of five minutes between topical applications in the same eye, or reflex tearing may wash out the first application. If possible hold the head of the animal flexed back for up to one minute after application so that more drug is absorbed by ocular tissues before draining through the nasolacrimal duct (to be absorbed systemically).

Dosages for intra-vitral injection of antibiotics in treatment of enophthalmitis. If performing intra-vitral injections it is of utmost importance not to damage the lens as this will lead to lens-induced inflammation

Drugs that are difficult to obtain in your country may be supplied by IDIS (www.idis.co.uk)

A good fortified topical antibiotic solution for use in the horse may be made as follows:

Nebcina (tobramycin) 4 vials of 40 mg in 1 ml: 160 mg/4 ml
Zinacef (cefuroxime) 250 mg disolved in 3 ml sterile water: 250 mg/3 ml
Serum (from centrifuge-spun blood taken from the horse) 5 ml
This will constitute a solution of
1.3% tobramycin + 2.1% cefuroxime + collagenase-inhibitors from the serum.
If the serum is spun in an EDTA-tube, EDTA's anti-collagenase action will be included in the solution.
This solution should be refrigerated and be discarded after 48 hrs and a new batch made up.

Drug	Dosage (up to)	Species
Ciprofloxacin	100–250 µgram	Rabbit
Gentamicin	100 µgram	
Cefazolin	2.25 mg	
Ceftriaxone	5 mg	Rabbit
Vancomycin	1 mg	

Name _____

i.d. _____

species _____

age/sex _____

history _____

adnexa

cornea

lens/anterior chamber

retina

Bibliography (compiled by T. Evans)

ACVO (1996). *Ocular disorders presumed to be inherited in purebred dogs*, Genetics Committee of the American College of Veterinary Ophthalmologists.

Barnett, A. (1990). *Color atlas of veterinary ophthalmology*. Wolfe.

Barnett, K.C., Crispin, S.M., Matthews, A. and Lavach, D. (1995). *Color atlas and text of equine ophthalmology*. Mosby-Wolfe.

Bodey, A.R. and Michell, A.R. (1996). Epidemiological study of blood pressure in domestic dogs. *J Small Anim Pract*, **37**, 116–125.

Bodey, A.R., Young, L.E., Barthram, D.H. et al. (1994). A comparison of direct and indirect (oscillometric) measurements of arterial blood pressure in anaesthetised dogs, using tail and limb cuffs. *Res Vet Sci*, **57**, 265–269.

Brooks, D.E., Andrew, S.E., Biros, D.J. et al. (2000). Ulcerative Keratitis caused by beta-hemolytic Streptococcus equi in 11 horses. *Veterinary Ophthalmology* **3**, 121–126.

Chambers, E.D. and Slatter, D.H. (1984). Cryotherapy (N_2O) of canine distichiasis and trichiasis: an experimental and clinical report. *J Small Anim Pract*, **25**, 647–659.

Chauvkin, M.J., Lappin, M.R., Powell, C.C. et al. (1994) Toxoplasma gondii specific antibodies in serum and aqueous humour of cats with experimental toxoplasmosis. *Am J Vet Res* **55**, 1244–1249.

Crispin, S.M. and Barnett, K.C. (1997). *Feline ophthalmology*. Saunders.

Dolowy, W.C. (1987). A safe, simple treatment for follicular conjunctivitis. *Vet Med*, 790–792.

Eisner, G. (1990). Eye Surgery. Springer-Verlag, New York.

Feenstra, R.P.G. and Tseng, S.C.G. (1992). What is actually stained by Rose Bengal? *Arch Ophthalmol*, **110**, 984–993.

Fischer, C.A. (1995). Ocular Feline Herpesvirus. A ten step approach to client communications. *Veterinary Forum*, 48–50.

Friedenwald, J.S. (1957). Tonometer calibration. *Trans Am Acad Ophthal Otol*, **61**, 108–123.

Frühauf, B., Ohnesorge, B., Deegen E. and Boevé, M. (1998). Surgical management of equine recurrent uveitis with single port pars plana vitrectomy, *Vet Ophthalmol*, **2**, 137–152.

Gaiddon, K., Kaswan, R.L., Hirsh, S.G. (1996) Radial keratotomy and third eyelid flap: Results of a novel approach to treatment of nonprogressive stromal ulcers and defects among dogs and cats. *Veterinary and Comparative Ophthalmology* **6**, 218–219.

Gelatt, K.N. (1978). *Veterinary ophthalmic pharmacology and therapeutics*. VM Publishing Inc, Bonner Springs, Kansas.

Gelatt, K.N. (1979). A modified subpalpebral system for the horse. *J Eq Med Surg*, **3**, 141–143.

Gelatt, K.N. (1999). *Veterinary ophthalmology*. 3rd edn. Lippincott, Williams and Wilkins.

Gerding, P.A. and Kakoma, I. (1990). Microbiology of the canine and feline eye.

Veterinary Clinics of North America. *J Small Anim Pract*, **20**, no. 3, May. Saunders.

Grant, R.L. and Acosta, D. (1994). Comparative toxicity of tetracaine, proparacaine and cocaine evaluated with primary cultures of rabbit corneal epithelial cells. *Exp Eye Res*, **58**(4), 469–478.

Helper, L.C. and Magrane, W.G. (1970). Ectopic cilia of the canine eyelid. *J Small Anim Pract*, **11**, 185–189.

Henik, R.A., Snyder, P.S. and Volk, L.M. (1997). Treatment of systemic hypertension in cats with amlodipine besylate. *J Am Anim Hosp Assoc* **33**(3), 226–234.

Kleinfeld, J. and Ellis, P.P. (1966). Effects of topical anesthetics on growth of microorganisms. *Arch Ophthalmol*, **76**, 712–715.

Lavach, J.D. (1990). *Large animal ophthalmology*. Mosby.

Lavach, J.D., Thrall, M.A., Benjamin, M.M. and Severin, G.A. (1977). Cytology of the normal and inflamed conjunctiva in dogs and cats. *J Am Vet Med Assoc*, **170**(7), 722–727.

Lawson, D.D. (1973). Canine distichiasis. *J Small Anim Pract*, **14**, 469–478.

Martin, C.L. (1999). Ocular manifestations of systemic disease. The dog. In: Gelatt, K.N. (ed.). *Veterinary ophthalmology*, 1401–1448. Lippincott, Williams and Wilkins.

Mattson, A., Roberts, S.M. and Isherwood, J.M.E. (1992). Clinical features suggesting hyperadrenocorticism associated with sudden acquired retinal degeneration syndrome in a dog. *J Am Anim Hosp Assoc*, **28**, 199–202.

Miller, P.E. and Pickett, J.P. (1992a). Comparison of the human and canine Schiotz tonometry conversion tables in clinically normal dogs. *J Am Vet Med Assoc*, **201**(7), 1021–1025.

Miller, P.E. and Pickett, J.P. (1992b). Comparison of the human and canine Schiotz tonometry conversion tables in clinically normal cats. *J Am Vet Med Assoc*, **201**(1), 1017–1020.

Miller, W.W. and Albert, R.A. (1988). Canine entropion. *Compendium of Continuing Education*. **10**(4), 431–438.

Nasisse, M.P., Guy, J.S. and Davidson, M.G. (1989). In vitro susceptibility of feline herpesvirus-1 to vidarabine, idoxuridine, trifluridine, acyclovir or bromovinyldeoxyuridine. *Am J Vet Res*, **50**, 158–160.

Nasisse, M.P., Guy, J.S., Stevens, J.B. et al. (1993). Clinical and laboratory findings in chronic conjunctivitis in cats: 91 cases (1983–1991). *J Am Vet Med Assoc*, **203**(6), 834–837.

Neer, T.M. (1984). Horner's syndrome: anatomy, diagnosis and causes. *Compendium of Continuing Education*, **6** (6), 740–746.

Olivero, D.K., Riis, R.C., Dutton, R.G. et al. (1991). Feline lens displacement. A retrospective analysis of 345 cases. *Prog Vet Comp Ophthal*, **1**, 239–244.

Peiffer, R.L., Gelatt, K.N. and Gwin, R.M. (1977a). Schiotz calibration table for the canine eye. *Canine Practice*, 49–51.

Peiffer, R.L., Gelatt, K.N., Jessen, C.R. et al. (1977b). Calibration of the Schiotz tonometer for the normal canine eye. *J Am Vet Med Assoc*, **38**(110), 1881–1889.

Prince, J.H., Diesem, C.D., Eglitis, I and Ruskell, G.L. (1960). *Anatomy and histology of the eye and orbit in domestic animals*. Charles C Thomas.

Quinn, A. (2000). *Corneal diseases in felines: treatments and comments*. Proc ASVO, April 2000, p. 17. Toronto.

Ramsey, D.T. and Fox, D.B. (1997). Surgery of the orbit. In: Nasisse, M.P. (ed.). Surgical management of ocular disease. *Veterinary Clinics of North America*. **27**(5), 1215–1264.

Ramsey, D.T., Hamor, R.E. and Gerding, P.A. (1995). Clinical and histological manifestations of extraocular polymyositis of dogs. *Trans Am Coll Vet Ophthalmol*, **26**, 37.

Schmidt, G.M. (1977). Problem oriented ophthalmology part 4: Corneal ulceration. *Mod Vet Pract*, 25–28.

Severin, G.A. and Thrall, M.A. (1981). Ocular exfoliative cytology. Proc 5th Kan Kal, 11–15.

Smith, P.J. (1999). Surgery of the canine posterior segment. In *Veterinary Ophthalmology*, ed by Gelatt, K.N., Lippencott, Williams and Wilkins, London 935–980.

Speiss, B.M., Wallin-Haakanson, N. (1999). Diseases of the Canine Orbit. In *Veterinary Ophthalmology*, ed by Gelatt, K.N., Lippencott, Williams and Wilkins, London, 511–534.

Spreull, J.S.A. (1966). Symposium: The Corneal Ulcer I. Anatomy and physiology of the cornea of the dog. *J Small Anim Pract*, **7**, 253–255.

Ugomori, S., Hayasaka, S. and Setogawa, T. (1991). Polymorphonuclear leukocytes and bacterial growth of the normal and mildly inflamed conjunctiva. *Ophthalmic Res*, **23**, 40–44.

Vainisi, S.J., Packo, K.H. (1995). Management of giant retinal tears in dogs. *Journal of the American Veterinary Medical Association* **15**, 491–495.

Van der Woerdt, A., Nasisse, M.P. and Davidson, M.G. (1991). Sudden acquired retinal degeneration in the dog: Clinical and laboratory findings in 36 cases. *Prog Vet Comp Ophthal*, **1**(1), 1–18.

Walde, I. (1990). *Atlas of opthlmology in dogs and cats*. B.C Decker Inc.

Whitley, R.D., McLaughlin, S.A. and Gilger, B.C. (1995). Update on eye disorders among purebred dogs. *Vet Med*, **90**, 574–592.

Wilkie, D.A and Whittaker, C. (1997). Surgery of the cornea. *Vet Clin North Am: Small Anim Pract*, **27**(5), 1067–1107.

Williams, D.L. (1994). Feline iridal disease – local and systemic implications. *Feline Practice*, **22**, 22–30.

Wills, M., Bounous, D.I. and Hirsch, S. (1997). Conjunctival brush cytology: evaluation of a new cytological collection technique in dogs and cats with a comparison to conjunctival scraping. *Vet Comp Ophthalmol*, **7**: 74–81.

Wolfley, D. (1987). Excision of individual follicles for the management of congenital distichiasis and localized trichiasis. *J Pediatr Ophthalmol Strabismus*, **24**(1), 22–26.

Index

Printed in the United States
By Bookmasters